LIVING
WITH
CANCER

CAROLINE ISADOR

KP PUBLISHING COMPANY

ISBN: 978-1-950936-61-8 (Paperback)
ISBN: 978-1-950936-62-5 (Ebook)
Library of Congress Control Number: 2020916875

Editor: Frank Williams
Cover Design: Juan Roberts, Creative Lunacy
Interior Design: Jennifer Houle
Literary Director: Sandra Slayton James

Published by:

KP Publishing Company
Publisher of Fiction, Nonfiction & Children's Books
Valencia, CA 91355
www.kp-pub.com

Printed in the United States of America

Dedication

I dedicate this book, firstly to the Triune God, without whom nothing is possible. Without His guidance and direction, I would have given up at the second chapter.

Secondly, to the two most influential women in my life, whose life stories, struggles and dreams for me, have been my inspiration:

My grandmother was a midwife, a fearless woman whose determination to create a legacy for herself, inspired my life.

My mother was a registered nurse, one of the first five nurses from our little hometown to graduate from University. Each night she would read stories to me of faraway lands and instill in me a desire to travel and expand my boundaries.

My mother was an avid believer in God and in His promise that, with Him "all things are possible." She died quite young in a tragic traffic accident, but she remains the lighthouse of my life.

Contents

SECTION 1: WHY ME?

SECTION 2: SURGERY AND RADIATION TREATMENTS

SECTION 3: LOOKING FORWARD WITH HOPE

SECTION 1
Why Me

THE INDENTATION

I remember, vividly, the first time I noticed the indentation. It was an unusually warm and still Friday evening last June; the air was almost stagnant. Not a branch swayed on any of the trees outside my complex. The usual ocean breezes were conspicuously absent as if nature was on the verge of heralding something unusual. I was toweling myself dry with my favorite fluffy, white oversized towel after having taken a long, cool shower.

As usual, during the warmer months, my shower always ends with a gradual decrease of hot water until it runs almost cold, allowing my body to feel refreshed and invigorated as the water temperature cools down. I was expected at a party at 8:00 p.m. and it was already 7:15 p.m. I always lose track of time when I am in the shower.

As I stood in front of the large bathroom mirror, I lifted my left breast, only to see what I would describe as an "indentation" at the bottom of the breast, just above where the breast rests on the rib cage. Staring into the mirror, I gently moved my fingers over and around the indentation several times. There was no pain, not even a sensation of any sort. I pressed a bit harder, but nothing. There was no discoloration or any difference in the texture of the skin near or around it. Although very puzzled, I continued to get ready for the party.

Three months later, I woke up to a bright Saturday morning in early September. I was pleasantly surprised that I had slept through the entire night with only one bathroom break. What a great feeling, one that has evaded me for quite a few years.

The only time during the past few years I had slept the entire night was on a visit to San Francisco. The hotel bed was just perfect, the mattress a medium firm, the pillows were like fluffy white clouds and the room completely black.

I will always remember that particular night because, before going to bed, I had sat out on the balcony for about an hour just savoring all of nature's sights and sounds. The sky was clear, the moon and the stars shone so brightly and appeared so close, it seemed as if I could almost reach out and touch one. I really enjoyed visiting San Francisco and hope to return one day.

This morning, I sauntered into my kitchen where the microwave clock displayed 7:45 a.m. This made me happy because I am usually awake by 6:00 a.m. each morning, even on weekends. I love early September mornings in Central Florida because, although the days are still quite hot, the early mornings are always pleasingly cool.

As I leaned against the kitchen counter, sipping a cup of green tea with honey, I looked outside the window through the space of the still missing pane of glass, which had popped out during the last hurricane and which I keep forgetting to have replaced, and noticed that fog had filled the air.

My reverie was interrupted by the scent of smoke drifting into my nostrils. The scent of smoke always unnerves me because as a child, our neighbor's home burned to the ground one quiet Saturday night as our family were all sitting at home listening to hits of the 60's and 70s on the radio.

At first, there were loud crackling sounds, then almost immediately the air was filled with the scent of smoke and sounds of people screaming. As fast as we were able to run outside to see what was happening, smoke and fire were billowing out of the back, corner windows of our neighbor's home. In just a few minutes after we got outside, the fire had spread to the roof and the acrid scent of different types of wood and shingles burning, took over the air. Then came the loud, popping sounds of pressurized containers of paints, oils, solvents and other chemicals exploding in the burning garage. All around us were the screams of neighbors shouting for everyone else to call the fire station. We did not have cell phones then, but a few of the neighbors had already called the fire station from their house phones.

Once it was established that no one had been left behind in the burning house, the women then concentrated on comforting the distraught homeowners and their children, while the men strenuously hosed down the neighboring homes to ensure no flying embers could cause the other roofs to catch afire. Although the fire truck came in just under seven minutes after the first call, in half an hour our neighbors had lost their entire home. It was completely heartbreaking for them and a horror for us to watch.

A pile of rubble now replaced their home. They were inconsolable and just stood there immovable; staring and crying, their bodies shaking. I will never forget the anguish and fear in the eyes of the children, with whom we walked to school each day. I never found out what caused the fire but it took almost nine months for them to rebuild and move back into the neighborhood. From that time on, the scent of smoke always triggers an alarm in my brain.

I am summoned back to reality and begin to take a much closer look around the condominium complex in which I lived, trying to determine from which direction the smoke scent was coming, but after a while it seemed to go away and I began to relax.

Still staring out of the window, I found myself, without thinking, rubbing the two middle fingers of my right hand under my left breast to feel if the "indentation" was still there or did it miraculously disappear overnight as I kept hoping it would. Although I initially decided, in June, not to worry about it, here I am now in September, standing in front of the kitchen window in my pajamas, watching the fog coming in off the ocean, and find myself reaching under my breast and realizing that, now months later, the little indentation is still there.

I go into the bathroom, unbutton my pajama top and look to see if it still appeared the same or if it had it deepened any more. It reminded me of an upside down, sucked inward triangular dimple. It was almost "cute" in its own way. I pressed it again, and again there was no pain or discomfort. Although I was not too worried, I decided to mention it to my primary care doctor when I went for my annual checkup in a few days' time.

Today is September 16th and I am waiting in the doctor's examination room, with only my underwear on and a sheet covering my body. I had two vials of blood drawn, earlier, from the little collapsible vein in my left arm. I heard my doctor coming down the corridor toward the exam room.

After the usual pokes, probes, stretches and taps, the questions begin. "Any concerns since your last visit?" he asked. I then raised up my left arm and lifted up the left breast and showed him the "indentation" He looked at it, rubbed his fingers over it and said in an offhanded manner, "Oh that's nothing to worry about Mrs. Isador, this *dimple* is not uncommon in many postmenopausal women. As long as there is no pain or change in its shape or color, you have nothing to worry about." "Thank you very much" I said with the biggest grin on my, now relieved, face.

I have the greatest respect for my doctor. He has been there for me over the years and has always worked miracles in bringing me through everything from simple personal rashes to stress-related problems, to bronchitis and more. If he says there is "nothing to worry about," then I will not spend another day worrying about it.

Every few weeks after the visit, however, I did a visual and self-examination to ensure there was no change in the size or look of the "dimple" and since there was no pain, after a while I forgot about it completely.

I decided to enjoy the last days of Fall, for what that is worth, in Florida. Fall brings in the most beautiful weather and it is the perfect time to go for daily, brisk walks to the beach and back. The coolness in the morning air and the light breeze provides a very pleasant change to the massive amount of humidity that is usually present in the Summer months.

In November, along with my three dearest friends, I went on a road trip down to the Florida Keys. To make the trip more exciting, we decided beforehand to do some research about the area and its history and settlement, so that when we arrived, we would be quite familiar with most of its landmarks as well as the culture. It was a long but very scenic trip down. We stopped twice during the drive for breakfast and lunch. We visited Key Largo, Marathon and Key West, where we spent three wonderful nights.

We were told by a tour guide that Ponce de Leon sailed north from the islands looking for the elusive Fountain of Youth which he never found, but he did come across the beautiful Florida Keys. The tour guide also told us a couple of stories about the Keys' discovery, but never verified the facts. It was all part of the fun.

The abandoned and existing bridges from South Miami to the Keys are a wonder to behold. Apparently, over the years there has been a total of 113 miles of roadway and 42 bridges connecting the Keys. They boast over two million visitors annually. Several large cruise ships were in the harbor the evening we arrived and Key West bustled with excitement and merriment. It was a great trip and we had an awesome time celebrating life with each other, capturing most of it on camera.

CHRISTMAS AND THE NEW YEAR

With my family and friends around me, I had a great Christmas. We ate, drank, and were very merry. I received some of the nicest gifts ever and was happy that I was able to give everyone on my list, the gifts I wanted for them. I was very upbeat. I was healthy and fit as a fiddle, thanks to my Jumba dance exercises. I had a healthy appetite for fun and life in general. I felt in tip top shape over the holidays and into the New Year.

The New Year dawned full of promise and I was ready to enjoy it to the fullest, asking God, of course, to bless me so that I could be a blessing to others.

It was in mid-February 2012 when my life took a curve and I began to experience discomfort at the bottom of my left breast, just where the bone of the bra rested on the rib cage. After two or three weeks, the discomfort began to really bother me so I discontinued wearing the "bone" bras and resorted to wearing the regular spandex ones (with no lift).

The discomfort, however, still did not go away to any acceptable extent, so on a trip to the city I went into one of the larger department stores, into the specialty area, and purchased a few of the very soft and flexible sports type bras and a few lace ones. I felt confident that the soft "boneless" bras would alleviate the discomfort under the breast area.

The new bras made no difference. A small wave of panic began to seep into my otherwise confident self. I stopped wearing bras altogether, whenever possible. It was now May and time for my annual mammogram, so I went and had the procedure done and a week later was advised that everything was normal. They explained that although there was the presence of some fibrous tissue in both breasts, there was no cause for concern. *Whew, I thought to myself, that surely is good news!*

A few days later, although still experiencing some discomfort and only being able to wear lace bras, the panic that had started to grip me before the mammogram, began to gradually fade away based on the positive news that my mammogram was "good."

Two weeks after the mammogram, however, the discomfort was replaced by a sharp pain just under and behind my left breast. I decided to go to the clinic of the local hospital. I explained my symptoms to the doctor who examined me.

"How long have you had this dimple under your breast?" she asked. "I noticed it back in June last year but my primary care doctor has assured me there is nothing to worry about and I have also just completed a 'good' mammogram."

Although a puzzled look quickly flashed across her face, she said nothing else about it. She diagnosed my condition as acute Gastroenteritis. I took the antacids she prescribed and felt quite relieved for about a week. I'm still unable to wear a regular bra, however, because the area continues to be extremely uncomfortable whenever the under strap of the bra touches it, but after taking the antacids the pain in my upper back, behind the left breast, subsided.

I was invited to a wedding and wanted to look young and pretty, so I endured the discomfort and wore a support bra because, not only would I be in close contact with the other guests, but I chose a close-fitting outfit, unlike the loosely fitted suits I wear at work. After a while, the pain became intense and distracting. I remained until the young couple's first dance and then scurried away. Immediately as I arrived home, I took off the bra and put a wet, cold towel over the area to try and ease the pain.

As a 56-year-old, I need the support a bra gives to my now, slightly sagging breasts. I feel that bras give outfits a "finished" look. Your clothes always seem to fit much better when wearing a good, supportive bra. Now that I am unable to wear a bra for any more than two hours at a time, I am no longer able to wear pullovers or snug fitting clothes. I have never had large breasts but I need all the support I could possibly get. As you can imagine, there is now a big shift in my wardrobe, to say the least, forcing me to wear suits or layered tops.

I am the Assistant to the Vice President of Marketing in a branch of a large, successful advertising firm and I am constantly in contact with staff as well as clients, so it has become quite a hassle to cover up this 56-year-old bra-less body and still look attractive.

I live alone in a large, comfortable, two-bedroom upstairs apartment in a complex in walking distance from the ocean and also not far from the heart of downtown of a very busy, but small town. I exercise regularly, well almost regularly, but I am better than most women my age in that regard. I am of medium/tall height and weigh 147 pounds.

I eat well, with only four days per week allowed for meat of any sort, and junk food is only allowed on Fridays which I refer to as my "Treat day." I get regular annual physicals and take care of my body as well as I know how.

I married young. When my dear husband died at only 38 years old, I had to bring up our children on my own, as best I could. Only one child did not finish college, and that was his choice, and he is paying for that choice now. Their ages range from 30 to 34; two daughters and one son. I also have four adorable, well balanced, grandchildren whom I love dearly. My children and grandchildren all live further north of here, about a three-hour drive by car. We visit a few times per year and we communicate by telephone, text and Skype almost daily.

I love my life. I have all the comforts I desire and although I do wish that I had saved more money over my lifetime for my swiftly approaching senior years, I have no major regrets. Most importantly, I am a devout Christian, and God is foremost in my life. I attend church twice weekly and I am part of our church's outreach program and other ministries.

I have a full life and although my extended family is quite small, I am surrounded by great friends from work, my old high school buddies and my church friends. I have an active social life which include church functions, work related activities, dinner parties and my closest friends and I get together on a regular basis to celebrate life.

I am not a complainer, so I have only mentioned my health concern regarding my breast/bra problem to my dearest friend. We are both baffled, especially as I have been cleared by three doctors and the mammogram has assured me that everything is fine.

Other than the "breast thing" I am very happy and healthy, especially as the "gas problem" that had caused me so much pain recently, has ceased almost entirely.

Three more weeks have passed. It is now the first day of August, and more than a year since I first discovered the dimple. The intense pain under the breast area is ongoing. I am also experiencing pain in the middle of my back, more to the left side, at the back of the rib cage.

So here I am again, sitting in the exam room of the hospital clinic, wearing a blue paper gown, clutching the back opening with my right hand, to keep it closed. I hear the doctor walking towards the door. It opens and I hear "Good morning Mrs. Isador, I see you are visiting us again." After explaining my symptoms, she diagnosed my latest problem as Costochondritis. She explained "It is an inflammation of the muscles around the chest/heart area." Armed with prescribed medication, I anticipated an imminent cure. I understood the diagnosis, because I had been diagnosed with the same condition some years back, I knew that in a week I would be feeling fine. I am, however, getting a bit tired of these, almost regular, doctor visits for the year so far.

Relief did come, but lasted only for about a week. The actual pain behind the breast area eased but the pain under the breast remained. A week later, the pain under the left breast intensified. That evening I went into the bathroom, removed my clothes and looked into the mirror. The dimple still looked the same. I began a closer examination of the area by slowly moving my fingers under and around the breast.

LUMPS

Are these lumps? I slowly rub my fingers under my breast again. I checked and rechecked. I moved my fingers along the bottom, sides and along every centimeter of my left breast. Panic overtook my whole being. I began to sweat and my head began to spin. I put a towel around me and went and sat on my bed.

Remember now, that over the past year, I have attended three doctors, including having a mammogram done and was told by each one that all was well. Except for the gastroenteritis and the costochondritis diagnoses, which I now realize could also have been misdiagnoses, each doctor assured me that everything was fine. My primary care doctor said that the dimple was not unusual, and the mammogram had shown nothing except some fibrous tissue, so these cannot be lumps I am feeling; only three months after the mammogram.

My first thought was that these are just lumps of fibrous tissue that are causing the pain, especially because the actual area of the lumps was not as painful. The excruciating pain was at the bottom of the left breast, right along the rib cage. I took a few very deep breaths and tried to calm down. I thought about it and decided that, rather than rush back to the doctors and complain again, after having been assured three times already that I was fine, I intentionally slipped into denial and decided to tolerate the pain and the very obvious lumps for a while longer.

Two weeks later and the pain is relentless, consuming my entire being. On the last day of August, a Thursday, eleven months after showing the dimple to my primary care doctor, and being assured that I had nothing to worry about, and three months after the "tumor free" mammogram, I called the radiologist whose office had performed the mammogram.

I described the pain and the lumps to her and insisted that, although the results from her office revealed that everything was fine with my breast, "something is definitely wrong" and I want her to personally and urgently review the mammogram results and revert as soon as possible.

After listening to me, she suggested that I come into the center immediately and she would have an ultrasound done. She explained that "the ultrasound might reveal images of the area that the mammogram may have missed"! What? "Missed?" Is that possible?

I am, once again, sitting in an examination room. The nurse asked me to remove all clothing above my waist and she placed a sheet over my body. The room is very cold and filled with large intimidating machines. The technicians came in and rubbed some type of gel over the area and then began the ultrasound scan.

The large machines were moved around until they loomed over my body, the breast area specifically. They then used a cup looking device and rolled it all over the breast. Click, click, snap, click went the machines. The technicians were both looking toward the monitor/screen that showed what was going on inside the breast. It only took a few seconds before a very dark, very dense looking mass showed up on the screen. I saw when the technicians looked at each other with very worried glances. I saw the mass and their reactions. I immediately knew that something was very wrong.

The male technician pointed to the mass and explained to me that it was about 2.5 cm wide. He began apologizing for not seeing anything when he did the mammogram three months earlier. He was very apologetic, but, as you can imagine, that meant nothing to me at this point in time, because it is now me, not him, that has been misdiagnosed and me, that now has a tumor in my breast.

I saw the male technician's eyes fill with tears, the reason for which, looking back now, I cannot really explain. He is the same technician who performed the mammogram three months earlier. Faced with a mass, which is obviously much more than three months old, he is most likely in fear of the consequences of his misdiagnosis. In all fairness, he should not be overly concerned because the doctor is just as culpable. She should complete an overview/verification and sign off on every diagnosis that the clinic performs (at least I would hope so). He pointed to the mass and explained what it was and what it meant. He then asked me to dress and he left the room.

Not long thereafter the door reopened and the nurse asked me to follow her. We walked out of the room and travelled along a long corridor to the (radiologist) doctor's office.

I could not "read" the doctor's facial expression. I imagine she had sufficient time to digest the information from the technician and brace herself for whatever I had to say with regards the misdiagnosis.

She tried to be upbeat and engaged in some chit chat, mixed with some information about her ordering an immediate biopsy. After about 10 minutes of nothingness in her office, I followed the nurse down the same long corridor to the same examining room I was in previously.

This time there was a team of three technicians waiting for me. The male technician who performed the ultrasound was in charge of the team. He mumbled something about the mass being in an area of the breast that was difficult for the machine to capture.

I can truly say, without any hesitation, that the next half hour's biopsy was the most painful procedure I have ever experienced. It was as if they were trying to squeeze the mass out of the breast through the nipple. The technicians were as rough as they could possibly have been. I wanted to scream out, at the top of my voice, in death squeals.

Delivering three seven-pound babies without painkillers, was a walk in the park compared to this biopsy. I had fractured my arm as a child, undergone eye surgery with minimal anesthesia, endured an appendectomy, hysterectomy and had my septum broken and reset. All of these together, were as nothing to compare with the level of pain I was presently experiencing. I have never endured two human beings, so violently, squeeze any part or portion of my body as these two technicians did, while the third one shoved an oversized "needle" into my breast. I wonder if they remembered to give me an injection of pain killers prior to the "crushing" to protect me from this violence. I cannot recall. I will never know.

They *stabbed* my breast with what appeared to be something similar to a Phillips Screwdriver. I felt as it went very deep into the core of the breast. These persons possessed herculean energy and strength.

It felt as if they were trying to pry my breast off my chest. By the time I left the clinic, I was so numb both physically and emotionally, I cannot remember anything I did or felt that afternoon or later that night. I was still in shock from being misdiagnosed, hearing the word "mass" being said to me and finally having the technicians stabbing my breast and seeming to crush it flat then pry it off my chest. It was entirely too much for me to bear. I do remember them advising the results would take seven days and they would call me at that time. The procedure left me completely breathless, and not in a good way. I was drained of everything good or positive.

CANCER

The word "Cancer" strikes terror into even the most calm and confident of individuals. I am quite certain that no one who has ever been diagnosed with cancer, just calmly walks out of the doctor's office and continues to proceed with their normal daily routine. Your mind immediately goes into a violent whirlwind of thoughts and fears. Nothing makes sense. All of those well thought out plans and dreams you had, seem to float away in one minute and during that minute, tomorrow seems so far away, actually, it feels as if tomorrow will never come.

Thoughts of death, sickness, suffering, financial ruin, loss of your career, your future, loss of everything that was real a few hours ago, invade your mind. You ask yourself,

> *"How soon will I become very ill?*
> *How many more months or years do I have?*
> *Can I possibly survive this?*
> *Who do I know who has survived the same cancer as I have?*
> *What will happen to my family?*
> *Who do I know who has died from this?"*

Your life, your mind, your future . . . it's all crushed and twisted. Right now, I feel like a delicate rag doll trapped in a ferocious tornado.

All these thoughts flood my mind as I am walking away from the diagnostic center toward my car. Whom do I tell first, whom do I tell at all? What do I say? Is this really happening to me? This all seems like a nightmare or a very scary movie. What about my family, what about my job, what about me?

WHY ME?

I eat right, I think. I exercise, I do not abuse drugs or alcohol. I am very careful to take vitamins and supplements. I think healthy thoughts. I am not overly stressed (I do not think so, anyway) and I take care of this "temple" that I call my body. "What have I done wrong, where did I go wrong?" I asked myself, "What has caused this horrible disease to invade my body?"

"Why me, why not one of those persons who hate life, or those perfectly healthy persons who commit suicide because, for one reason or the other, they hate their life and everything about it.

Why not one of those persons who walk the streets wishing they were dead? What about all the sexual and physical abusers, the horrible predators, the soulless rapists?

What about all the murderers who have no respect for life? Why not them? Why do they seem to live full healthy long lives?

Why me? WHY? Why innocent children, why anyone?" Most likely I will never find the answers to these questions. So, I will not waste any more valuable time worrying.

In Psalms 139:16 it states that God knew us before we were born and each day of our lives is planned out and recorded in His book, so, while this is a surprise to me, it is not a surprise to God. I am sure His plans and His will for my life are wonderful, so I will leave the "Why Me" to Him as much as is humanly possible.

So, what now? Well, I guess I get into to my car, leave the center's parking lot and try to decide whether to go home and call my family or wait for the biopsy results. "What, what, what do I do now?"

I drove to the nearest fast food restaurant I could find and bought a large chicken sandwich combo with a large fruity, sugary drink. I then drove home, sat down and ate the meal.

As I ate, I remembered something that I read some time back and it said that life does not always go the way we feel it should, but rather it is just the way it is. However, the way we cope with it, is what makes the difference, so I tried to focus on God and His promises versus what now felt like an impending death sentence.

Twenty-four hours later, what had been a relatively perky, pink left breast was now a bruised, deep purple mass of pain and suffering. The massive crushing my breast had undergone at the hands of the technicians during the performance of the biopsy, had left a swollen, bruised piece of horribly discolored, sick looking flesh on the left side of my chest.

I feel like a zombie. Even though I am trying to be positive, fear has overtaken my every thought, my entire day, and my perspective on life. Simultaneously, I am fiercely trying to hold on to my faith and God's promises.

I have not yet told anyone. I do not know what to say, after all, the "mass" had not yet been officially labeled. Looking back, I realize that I went to work the day following the ultrasound and biopsy and despite the intense pain, with the help of some strong painkillers, performed to my usual high standard.

I was cheerful and helpful and spoke to my children with the usual witty demeanor—but all the time I was in purgatory—just hanging on to my daily routine and barely breathing, not even allowing myself to think. I did not know what to think about so I just existed, with the word "mass" ringing over and over in my head. Thank goodness for the weekend ahead, when I could be alone.

I was told I had to wait for seven business days to hear my fate. I never knew that seven days could take such a toll on me or that time would move along so slowly. It was as if time just stood still. When the seventh day came and passed and I did not receive a call, I was too afraid to pick up the phone and call the clinic.

It was not until another four days had passed that my primary care doctor called. "Can you come in to see me as soon as possible, preferably today?" I found out later that he thought that the diagnostic clinic had called me and they thought that, because they had sent the results to him, that he would call me.

Another screw up!! He did not initiate this test, in fact, according to his last words to me, I had "nothing to worry about" so I see no reason why the results were sent to him. Unless, of course, the doctor (radiologist) did not wish to face me with the news that her clinic had screwed up.

I cannot imagine how many hundreds of thousands of persons are in the grave today because of medical screw ups, mistakes and misunderstandings.

My doctor's face seemed, in that moment, to have aged years. I wonder if he was remembering/acknowledging to himself, that he had misdiagnosed me. He was the one who advised that the inverted triangle under my breast was "not unusual in menopausal women. There is nothing to worry about." In any event, as I had expected, he did not acknowledge any memory of that fateful visit; not even the slightest acknowledgement thereof.

He began speaking in an ominous voice and gently pushed the biopsy results over the desk towards me and asked me to read the report. I did. I was very calm. No, actually, I only appeared to be calm, I was not calm, not calm at all. I was experiencing the lack of any emotion except shock and awe, with a side of total panic and fear.

My earlier conclusions were definitively confirmed by the report in front of me. I had seen the word "Cancer" hundreds of times, but never on the same piece of paper with my name at the top of it.

He eventually, very slowly, retrieved the piece of paper from me. I maintained my silence. "Do you understand what these results mean?" "I do" I said. However, it was as if he did not believe that I had read it, or maybe he felt I misunderstood what it contained. He proceeded to read it aloud, very quietly and solemnly. He asked, "do you realize that there is cancerous tumor in your left breast?"

I whispered, "I fully realize what is happening." At that moment, I felt as if all the blood in my body had drained out of me. My feet became very heavy. My breathing became labored. I was just an empty vessel with this "strange" person sitting and talking at me.

He shared some information about cancer, the seriousness thereof and the options, etc., none of which I heard or even cared about, for that matter. He wrote up some referral forms and continued to speak. He called his nurse in and gave her some instructions. I continued to hear nothing he was saying. Eventually my mind and thoughts returned to the moment and I rose up from the chair, took the forms and followed the nurse to the nurses' station.

"We are referring you to a very reputable surgeon at the best hospital in the area" she said. The appointment was for three days later. I truly cannot remember what I did when I left the doctor's office. I do not recall anything of the next couple of days. I knew I had to tell my children.

TELLING MY CHILDREN

I rehearsed over a hundred times what I would say to my children and nothing felt right. My dilemma was compounded by the fact that, just two days prior, my oldest daughter had called crying and saying that she was quitting her job the following day. She discussed it with her husband and they both agreed. "Mum, the stress is unbearable," she wailed. "I am physically and emotionally unable to cope another day without having a nervous breakdown." She added that although she had no prospects of any job opportunities at the time, she had no choice but to leave immediately.

With that stress in mind and without any prepared speech, I asked God's guidance to help me. I decided to do a conference call to all three children. I began by saying that I had something important to discuss with them and that I did not want them to interrupt until I was finished. Deadly silence from them all. As you can imagine, none of them could have predicted what I was about to say.

I tried to simplify the whole thing as much as possible and also remain as calm and upbeat as possible, ending my discourse with, "the prognosis is excellent so there is nothing to really worry about. The 'stage' has not yet been determined, but the surgeon will perform more tests during the surgery to determine that aspect of it."

Again, deadly silence. Eventually my son said, "Mum, I am sure everything will be just great." I was not surprised at his comment because that is how he removes himself from any stressful situation or responsibility of consequence, by announcing that "everything will be just great." His comment triggered an outburst from the girls. They, of course, did not share the same perfect prognosis as he did. "This is not the time for arguments," I said. The girls then began to ask questions and I answered to the best of my ability, remaining as calm as possible.

My oldest daughter said that she would drive down to be with me during the surgery and stay until she felt comfortable that I was able to cope by myself. Although I was grateful and happy that she was able to be with me during the surgery and beyond, it did bring to mind the fact that she only had the available time because she was now unemployed. The other siblings advised they would all come down on the Friday evening after the surgery to spend the weekend with me. I looked forward to seeing them.

I then called my Pastor who, along with two elders in the church, promised to come by that same evening to pray with me. Finally, I called my best friend and told her, "Call me when your Pastor leaves and I will bring you supper and we could share our feelings about this whole thing." I am sure she needed to hear it again as she, obviously, did not accept what she "just heard." We later had a nice meal but she was in such an emotional state, I ended up comforting her.

The following day I met with the head of Human Resources and my boss. I explained to them that I was scheduled to have a" feminine" surgery and would be off from work for about four to six weeks. I decided that was enough information to share at the moment. Because my boss is also my friend, I would have to tell her soon. But, not now.

I did not want a pity party, neither did I want them to share the information (in secret) with anyone else in our small office. When I needed to provide more details, as time went on, I would. I promised to bring in the "Sick Certificate" from the doctor within a few days.

My next memory was of walking into the surgeon's suite a few days later. Here I am, again, sitting in an examination room, with a paper gown on, this one being white. My blood pressure was being taken, my weight and dozens of health questions were being asked. I then dressed and was escorted down a corridor towards the surgeon's office.

I remember trying to be upbeat; however, I was sitting in front of another drawn, solemn face looking into mine. Many times, the look on the faces of the doctors' make the whole process even more ominous. While he continued to look over the notes, I tried making small talk, but was interrupted by his slipping the same Report towards me, just as the previous doctor had done.

This must be some official procedure when cancer is being discussed. "Please read this and tell me what you feel." Was he joking? What did he mean, "Please tell me what you feel?" I felt like slapping his face with a 10-pound mallet. I felt like causing bodily harm to the doctors who had misdiagnosed me. I felt very angry, very hurt and very scared and at the same time I felt empty and confused.

I totally believe in God's will for my life, but, at the same time, my whole being is trying to come to grips with why? why this?? Why now? and again, I try to calm myself with the big picture, God's promise to me that He would never leave me or forsake me IF I have complete faith in Him and His will and promise for my life; however, my faith is very difficult to hold on to at this moment.

I looked the surgeon directly in his eyes. I said, "I totally understand the diagnosis, but with so many different emotions going on in my head, I do not know if I am able to clearly express myself." "Take a deep breath and take your time," he said. He was very gentle.

I began slowly. "I believe in God's will for my life and accept that everyone on earth has an entrance date and an exit date and it is the quality of life in between those times that create one's legacy." I continued, "I did not create myself and neither did I have the specifications for the time frame of my existence. I have lived a very good life, a full and happy life and while stained with the sad memory of my husband's untimely passing, life has been kind to me so far." I said, "If it is God's will, I would love to live at least another twenty more healthy years and make more memories with my family and friends, but if it is not His will, then so be it, my life and my future are in His hands.

My hope, if this condition becomes terminal, is not to push the envelope and spend every penny I have sacrificed so many years to save, on experimental medicine and unnecessary surgeries and then eventually, when I could no longer pay for the 'care', be forced to endure horrible debilitating pain and suffering and eventually die helpless, bitter, broken, and penniless.

I do not wish to leave this earth a comatose, bedridden, hollowed out shell whose last months and last funds were spent contributing to the egos and ambitions of emotionless medical research personnel. I wish to be spared that."

I explained that while I do believe in and applaud modern medicine, I do not wish to be a guinea pig or some experimental rat contributing to the furtherance of science and making already rich doctors and big Pharma, even richer through unnecessary "treatments" and procedures.

I ended by saying, "If I were to get really sick from this disease, I wish, at that time, to be allowed to maintain my respect and to keep my dignity. I would want to be treated with mega dose pain killers, and let nature take its course. I want to slip away into my next existence as quietly and as peacefully as possible to join my family and friends who have gone ahead of me into glory." I said, "I am of the firm conviction that I will worship God equally, despite the outcome."

It was obvious that, on no level, was he was prepared for my response. Well, he had asked how I felt, had he not? Now he knows exactly how I feel. Actually, my long discourse made me feel much better, especially because he did not interrupt or change his facial expression, so I was able to get it all out.

He sat for a long time, just pulling on his beard and looking down at his desk. After a while, he slowly lifted his head and as his eyes met mine, he said "You are a very strong-willed woman. I totally understand and respect your feelings and I admire your resolve." His demeanor then lifted considerably and he began discussing what "we" needed to do next. "Let's have the PET CT scan done today." He had his nurse call to confirm the surgery could be done the following Wednesday morning. She called back within a few minutes and said that it was booked for 7:30 a.m.

He discussed chemotherapy and radiation treatments and I told him that although I would agree to undergo the radiation treatments, I do not wish to have any chemotherapy medicine enter my body. We went into further discussion about my choices and after much back and forth, he got me to agree to, at least, speak with a medical oncologist to learn more about the latest strides in modern cancer treatments.

He then drew a detailed diagram of the breast and very carefully explained how he intended to remove the mass. Because of where the tumor was located, rather than remove the entire breast, he intended to surgically remove a triangular section of the breast from the nipple down to the very bottom, where the breast skin meets the rib cage, ensuring all of the mass is removed and then pull together and stitch the remaining portion of the breast.

"The procedure is called a Lumpectomy, and although the report from the diagnostic center states that the cancer had not spread to the lymph nodes, I will examine and take samples of the lymph nodes near the breast during the surgery, to ascertain if the cancer has, in fact, seeped into them."

To do this, he advised, he would have to perform a surgical incision under the armpit area as well. It would require a straight line cut to access the nodes. If it appears cancer is present, he would remove all diseased nodes and surrounding tissue. He summed up by stating that the whole procedure should take no more than three hours, maximum, and that I should be awake shortly afterwards. I left his office much more confident and knowledgeable about what to expect. I decided I liked him, respected him and trusted him.

Surgery and Radiation Treatments

THE SURGERY

I returned to the hospital two hours later to have the PET-CT scan done. The abbreviation PET-CT means Positron Emission Tomography and is a nuclear medicine imaging technique that produces a three-dimensional image of functional processes in the body. This process provides detailed pictures of tissues and organs inside the body and reveals any abnormal activity that might be going on inside.

To facilitate the scan, a small amount of radioactive substance is injected into a vein, and as well, I had to drink a large amount of a chalky tasting fluid. The substance is absorbed mainly by organs and tissues that use the most energy. Because cancer cells use more energy than healthy cells, they absorb more of the radioactive substance. A scanner then detects this substance to produce pictures of the inside of the body.

The whole process was not as frightening as I thought it would be. I had imagined a coffin like procedure, but it was an open procedure in which a dome, of sorts, moves up and down over the entire body for about forty-five (45) minutes. You have to lie completely still during the entire process, hardly even a blink of an eye is allowed. I was amazed to realize they were taking images from the tippy top of my head to the bottom of my big toe.

Afterwards they suggested that I drink lots of water, in order to eliminate, from my body, the substance that was ingested earlier. Afterwards, I was given a DVD and a written report of the entire procedure to pass along to my doctor.

My daughter arrived the evening prior to the surgery and the following morning at 7:00 a.m. we arrived at the hospital. I checked in at the front desk and was directed to the pre-op area. At 7:30 I was on the operating table being prepped for the surgery.

The anesthesiologist, the operating team, the technicians and nurses were all scurrying around, taking my vitals, x-rays, blood work and sharing information about what I could expect during and immediately after the surgery. They were very efficient. I was signing permission forms and listening to them as they "prepped" me for the surgical procedure.

My surgeon then came in. "How are you feeling?" "I am feeling quite well," I assured him. The anesthesiologist enquired whether I preferred an injection to "put me to sleep" or to have the mask placed over my nostrils and mouth, I preferred the injection. As I lay there looking around the room, it occurred to me that the lighting in the operating theatre was very dim and I remembered noticing the same thing, the last time I had had surgery. I imagine it must be to highlight the lighting from the very bright spotlights that are turned on during the surgery.

Just about three hours later, I heard the nurse calling my name. I opened my eyes and realized that it was all over and I was awake. I felt no pain at the time, just a bit of soreness and tightness around the area that was operated on.

Everything had gone very well. My surgeon came by early the following afternoon and was pleased with how I tolerated the surgery. Armed with specific care instructions, I was allowed to go home later in the day. I was given an arm sling to wear on my left arm for the next five days, to ensure I did not move the arm unduly, which could cause the stitches to break, or worse.

I was given six weeks off from work to ensure my healing and recovery would be maximized. My daughter drove me home and promised to stay with me until my first check up or until she was confident that I could manage on my own. My best friend met us upon our arrival home, with a large bouquet of flowers and a fruit bowl and assured my daughter that she would check on me twice daily after returning home. My daughter was very relieved. She prepared a light meal for us and an hour later, I was asleep.

I followed the doctor's instructions very carefully and was very mindful not to wet the bandages or move my arm in any way that would "pull" the skin under my armpit where the lymph nodes incision had been made, or the breast area, which had had a significant portion removed. A couple days later, the skin around the breast area and under the armpit, began to feel "stretched" as if someone was tugging at it from both directions. I got accustomed to keeping the arm very still to avoid any accidents.

By the fourth day, I had had enough of bed and decided to go out and enjoy a bit of sun. It was after all, the third weekend in September and the heat was not as intense. With my arm still in the sling, we took a slow walk around the complex and the sun did a great deal of good for my mood and my recovery. The light sea breeze filled my lungs with peace and hope. The pain was not unbearable, although, I was still quite medicated, but not groggy.

The first week went by faster than I thought it would, quite possibly because my daughter was there to keep my spirits up and take care of me. We shared how alike as well as how different we both were. The other siblings and my grandchildren arrived the Friday night and spent the weekend pampering me. We were all very happy the surgery went well and they were amazed at how well I looked.

FIRST FOLLOW UP VISIT

The following Wednesday I was again sitting in my surgeon's office, this time for my first post-op check-up. My daughter accompanied me. She wanted to ensure

I was well enough before she returned home to her family and begin some serious job hunting.

I am in the, now familiar, examination room, this time in a colorful cloth gown. The doctor walks in, with the usual somber expression. I determined to change the mood he was bringing into my space, so I came up with some silly anecdote and it worked. A slight smile creeped over his, otherwise somber, but handsome face. "The surgery went quite well. The lab results show that the cancer has reached Stage 2, T2 (2.5cm) N1 (1/2) MO. The tumor was just under one inch and had spread to three axillary lymph nodes, but had not metastasized further."

He removed the bandages and appeared pleased with his work and my healing so far. "Continue to take the prescribed medicine, take it easy for the next few weeks and ensure the wound area is properly cared for." He told me that if I had any concerns to call him. He then made an appointment for me to return the following week for another examination of the incision. "I took a sample of the breast tissue (removed during the surgery) and sent it off to have some receptor studies done to determine if you are a candidate for hormone therapy."

We again discussed chemotherapy and radiation. I agreed to the radiation treatments, but I reminded him that I did not wish to subject my, already compromised, body to chemotherapy. Despite what we discussed at our previous pre-surgery meeting, he again suggested I visit a medical oncologist in the city. I told him that I prefer seeing someone locally. The doctors at the large, well known facilities in the city charge a great deal more than the local doctors because they are all renowned specialists and consultants.

Another week has passed and my daughter is back with her family. Before she left, she prepared and froze many meals for me for the following week. She also went grocery shopping and purchased everything I could possibly need in the near future. I am so thankful that she was able to be with me during and post-surgery. I assured her that I had every confidence that she would find employment very shortly, because she was very skilled in her profession.

Although a bit painful and uncomfortable at times, I am feeling much stronger and more confident with the progress of the healing of my breast and the incision under my armpit. I push myself a little more each day to regain my pre-surgery mobility and routine.

Each morning I take a short walk around the complex and then prepare a light healthy breakfast. My breast feels heavy when I walk, so I wear sports tops, under my blouse so that the breast does not jiggle about. Of course, I cannot wear bras yet. I cup the breast in my hand when I get up through the night to use the bathroom.

My best friend calls early each morning to check on my needs and brings me dinner each day, after work. On the weekends she assists with cleaning, laundry and some bulk meals. She also does my grocery shopping. She is a life saver. My daughters, without their families, drove down at the end of the second week and did everything that needed to be done. That gave my friend a weekend break. They brought so much grocery, I felt as if a hurricane was on its way and we were told to stock up. They were very relieved to see that I was able to move around so well and was in high spirits.

It is now four weeks post-surgery and I have returned to my doctor to check on the wound and its progress. He was pleased with the healing process and this time he seemed in a particularly good mood. He said I must return in 10 days' time; no more weekly visits.

Three days short of six weeks post-surgery, my surgeon announced that I am now able to return to work. He suggested my next step be to speak with the radiation oncologist. He instructed his staff to make all of the necessary arrangements for me to see her as soon as possible. He said, "This radiation oncologist is very well respected, having worked in Canada and New York before moving to Florida and I am pleased to recommend her to you."

Returning to work was a big confidence booster and my co-workers, some of whom had visited me after the surgery, were very welcoming and helpful the first few days until I got back into my routine. Except for my left arm being a bit stiff because I had babied it for the past six weeks, which slowed my typing down a bit, everything fell back into place quite nicely.

I was still unable to wear a bra and finding blouses, in my closet, that were non-abrasive, was a new challenge. Even though I wore the sports tops, they did not cover the armpit area where the scar from the lymph nodes was still healing. Any abrasive fibers irritated it.

A week later I found myself sitting in an office which was quite run down, virtually bare of any decoration or any hint of an attempt to make it pleasing to the eye. I was sitting in front of an old, worn down desk that, I was sure, has paid for itself many times over. Behind the desk, however, sat a very pretty, pleasant, but serious young female radiation oncologist. She appeared to be confident in her craft and we got right down to business.

She read the notes that had had been sent to her by my surgeon, as well as the PET-CT scan report and explained in careful detail, the surgery that had been performed on my breast. She detailed exactly what the dimensions of the mass (tumor) meant. She drew diagrams of the specifics of where the tumor was in relation to the rib. "Do you realize that the tumor was less than a centimeter away from the bone?" She then explained what this could mean going forward and suggested that I begin radiation therapy immediately. Inside of me, I screamed,

"Dear God, what does this mean?
Please God do not let this scourge go into my bones"
Inside I was screaming as loud as my inner voice would allow.
"Do not let this seep into my bones, please God! Please God, this has already
spilled into the lymph nodes, please do not let this go into my bones—
I beg of you, dear Father God, I need you to make this miracle happen in
my body and my life right now!"

On the outside, I tried to appear calm while she called the team leader at the radiation center and asked when would be his first available opening. I was to see him in two weeks. She also prepared the notes for me to take to the head technician at the radiation center.

We spoke for at least an hour, she was very honest and upfront—she explained the possibilities, the costs, she cited examples of other patients she tended to and their various conditions and outcomes. I told her I was a Christian and believed in God. She confirmed that she, too, was a Christian.

She was a bit disappointed I was alone for the initial consultation because so much information is covered, it would have benefitted me to have someone help absorb everything and assist afterwards with recollection of the details.

What impressed me most about this young doctor was when, nearing the end of our discussion, she said "I'm a firm believer in God and His will for all of us. I ask for His involvement in everything I put my hands to. In my experience, how the patient progresses, depends to a great extent on his/her spirituality, their frame of mind, faith in God and belief in themselves to overcome this battle of healing, and courage, no matter how it turns out."

She believed that our earthly life is only a small portion of our full existence and once we believe that God's will for our lives is perfect, we then continue "healing" whether it is physical or spiritual or both. She said that after such a life changing experience, life would never be the same again.

As expected, she also suggested chemotherapy in addition to the radiation treatments. She advised that the course of radiation could cost upwards of $20,000 which would include the weekly consultations with the doctor and oncologist visits. She really impressed me, and I felt totally comfortable in her presence. But it is amazing that after an hour of consultation, only one sentence remained in my head: "The tumor was less than a centimeter away from the bone"

Despite her insistence, I opted against the chemotherapy but agreed to begin the six-week period of daily radiation therapy. I valued her suggestion regarding the chemo, but assured her that I would take full responsibility for my decision not to poison my body with the chemotherapy chemicals.

I will undergo the radiation treatments, and radically change my thought process, by completely placing my life in God's hands and ask that His perfect will be done in my life. I, personally, do not accept that poisoning my "temple" will heal me. I transferred my trust from the earthly doctors to "the Great physician, God" to lead me through this challenge of cancer.

The first thing I did was to ask God to show me what, if anything, I was doing wrong or thinking wrong and to lead me to healthy lifestyle habits, healthy eating habits, healthy thinking (all of which I totally believe, are inter related) and more than anything, I asked His guidance in how to please Him.

Before I left her office, she explained that the radiation treatments consist of five weeks of specific radiation treatment to the entire left breast and lymph node area under the left armpit. The sixth week would entail a period of higher dosages of radiation and more specific targeting of the lymph nodes, the area of the breast that housed the tumor and the area where the breast touched the rib cage.

During the first week after the surgery and recovery, I had done a great deal of thinking and praying. Prayer is a very important part of my life and I believe with all my heart that prayer, in accordance with God's will for us, is heard and answered. I totally believe that God is the Great Physician and that the surgery was guided by Him and performed by my doctor. I pray earnestly and often, asking my Creator to guide me along this journey.

Reminder: *"More things are wrought by prayer than this world dreams of."*
Lord Tennyson.

This is a totally unexpected turn in my life. As you may imagine, I vacillate between bouts of confusion and uncertainty, even doubt at times. I constantly need to be redirected back into His word and His will for this journey of mine, called life. I am convinced that this experience is taking me from one level of life to another completely different level—one from which I will emerge a much more faithful, trusting, hopeful and joy filled person, no matter what the outcome.

Before this experience, I continually worried about my future financial position and whether or not I was going to have enough money saved with which to retire comfortably. My health was the last thing on my mind. I felt completely healthy and confident that once I did what I should do; eat right and exercise, everything would be just fine, especially as there was no history of cancer in my family (as far as I am aware).

Now, I truly believe that all I need is God. He can do everything in and through whomever He wishes for me and I made a conscious decision to direct my life toward more prayer. I have asked God to keep my knees strong so that I could kneel each night before I retire to bed, to thank Him for bringing me safely and healthy through the day.

I thank God for allowing me to be a blessing to others and to allow others to see His light in my life. I ask His forgiveness for the things I do during each day that does not please Him and I ask His guidance for the day ahead. I ask for healing, His strength and His mercy. I ask Him to bless those I love and those with whom I may come in contact with the following day. I then ask Him to bless those persons in my church and in my circle of friends who are in need of prayer and healing, as well as my colleagues and the company I work for.

MY CHILDHOOD/SPIRITUALITY

I was a happy child, in fact, every picture of me shows me with a huge grin on my face. I grew up totally oblivious to what was happening in the outside world. It was vastly different from nowadays. We played outback of our house and went to neighbors' homes to play with their kids and when our parents wanted us, they went outside and shouted really loudly and we came running back home.

We rode our bicycles blocks away from home without any fear or trepidation of predators or any harm of any kind. We rode down hills with our hands up in the air, with no thought that a car may side swipe us or that the bicycle may hit a bump or a rock and we could spin out of control.

The kids on our street all walked to and from school together and although there was the occasional scuffle, it was not carried to the next level of "serious" or anything like that. We all stood in a circle and watched every fight that took place. Whoever won the fight won the argument and we all then proceeded home together.

As a child, I daydreamed a great deal. Most of my daydreams centered around my growing up and having a family and a beautiful home. I dreamed that me and my husband would travel the world for the first few years and then settle down and have a beautiful Cape Cod home and a large happy family. I had vivid mental pictures of how my living room would look. I remember that my dreams displayed the room with white walls and red and black furnishings.

For those of you in your late 50s and 60's, you may remember the animal patterns and the reds and blacks that were the "in colors" in those days. I also pictured a round bed with fluffy bedspreads and sheepskin throw rugs all around the bed.

By the time I married and eventually owned a home, those colors were no longer in style, neither were round beds or sheep skin throw rugs, but I still recall the pictures in my mind's eye. I also pictured a small vegetable garden in the back yard with a large tree in the center of the yard, from which would hang a swing for my children and hopefully for my grandchildren. I planned to have pretty flowers all along the perimeter of my yard and others hanging from the large trees that I intended to plant.

When I met and married my best friend, I never ever thought I would be a widow and a single mother at such a young age, and as if that were not enough, I never thought I would eventually be faced with breast cancer, and Stage 2 to boot!!

Since my youthful dream days, I have:

experienced the bliss of a happy marriage,

the joy and blessing of giving birth to three healthy and happy children,

the life altering loss of my dear husband,

having to raise our three children on my own,

having to sell the marital home in order to help pay college fees for my children,

having to relocate into a two-bedroom condominium,

going back to school (College) to get the degree I never got before I married

and here I am now, facing the biggest challenge of my life so far.

The first question I asked myself when I was diagnosed was "Do you believe that you will survive this?" I immediately went to the Bible for a possible response, even before I told my family. I studied what God had to say about sickness, sin, healing, faith and the life hereafter. After all, He is the Great Physician, and He is also the One who created us and provided the manual (the Bible) for our lives so I felt it was the only sensible thing to do, to firstly seek His guidance and wisdom.

After much prayer and study, I then asked myself, "How much effort are you willing to put into this to be able to push past the doubts, the negative diagnoses, the pain and the suffering?" I reminded myself of what Jesus did for me and why, and decided to rely on God's promises laid out in the Bible. I continued to read and fully accept that God sacrificed His only son in order that we may have life and have it more abundantly. Jesus gave His life so that we can have our sins forgiven and our diseases healed (according to God's will for our lives) so I am trying to discover what God's will is for my life. I tried to dig deep, very deep to see if, at all possible, I could figure out WHY God allowed this disease to visit my life.

I then realized that only constant study, prayer, and meditation could possibly enlighten me to the answers to these questions (if ever, fully). I made a commitment to believe and follow what I had read in the bible and what my Christian upbringing had instilled into me.

Firstly, I thanked God that the cancer had only reached Stage 2—it could have been so much worse. I know friends who were already at Stage 4 by the time they were diagnosed. I realize that God is allowing me to fully experience and understand this disease, so that I would have to rely completely and totally on Him and His word and promises for my life and not go around telling others (if I survived) what I, Caroline, did to survive. Instead, my story would be **what God did** to save my life, according to His will for me.

I thank Him for my life, my family, my job, His mercy toward me and those I love. Most of all I ask forgiveness for whatever I have willingly and unknowingly done to displease Him. Over the past weeks, I spent many hours thinking of persons I may have offended, angered or insulted and I asked forgiveness, specifically including the names of those I had knowingly offended. I went to the extent of calling and writing to some persons asking their forgiveness.

It was of paramount importance to me, to ensure my life was pleasing to God and that I had no ill will toward anyone or held any bitterness, anger or unforgiveness in my soul because it is common knowledge that these negative traits can sometimes be the root causes of many diseases, heart attacks, strokes and other stress related disease. In other words, I am on a mission to do my best to clean house, my soul's house.

Life lesson: It starts with me . . .

You may think this is extreme, but this was my personal decision and, in each instance, I was met with very positive responses from those I called and two, to my delight, looked forward to resuming our friendships. Surprisingly, in the other two instances, I actually received heartfelt apologies for their part in our rift. I felt so free. I can barely explain it. I had also read in the Bible that I should go before the elders of my church and ask for their prayers for healing, which I did. Nowhere, however, did I read that I had to go and tell all my friends and co-workers, so I decided to just stay in prayer and only tell persons who, I felt, at this time absolutely needed to know, which, of course, eventually included two persons at work in the Human Resources department (who would see all the large Insurance bills coming in and would realize that something "big" was happening with my health). Because of their positions, I trusted them to respect my privacy. I had told my peers that I had some personal feminine health issues that required surgery.

Thankfully, I would be able to undergo the radiation treatments during my lunch hour, because the cancer center is just four blocks from my office and the procedure only takes 30 minutes.

I kept reading God's promises to me, especially Psalms 103 which tells me that God forgives all our sins and that He is still in the Healing business, along with other scriptures including Philippians 4:6 which always give me hope to continue any struggle, knowing that God has promised me that this battle is His own, not mine to worry about. It is between Him and the Evil one, Satan. I decided to hold God to His word, I decided to obey Him and leave all the consequences to Him, as Dr. Charles Stanley would say. I have seen persons who were diagnosed with cancer and within two weeks had told everyone they knew, only to discover that 90 per cent of those they told were either negative about their chances for recovery or were pitying the patient and the problem.

It is my firm belief that when faced with any life-threatening challenge, you need to be as positive as possible. Announcing your problem to "the world" hardly ever gets you the positive support you need to move ahead. Pity parties usually result in second guessing your chances and placing an over-emphasis on your symptoms and the disease. What you need at a time like this is to forge ahead with your healing and only "regurgitate" each step of the way to a small, necessary, group of persons.

Often times when persons, who are aware of your challenge, question how you are doing, you find yourself repeating the whole process of treatment, pain, details of surgery and how the breast is healing, etc. again and again, and after a while you hear yourself speak of so much "sickness" you convince yourself that you are actually sicker than you really are. That, of course, is my personal opinion and experience.

The more persons treat me as healthy and normal, the healthier and more normal I feel and that is how I have survived thus far in life. When asked how I am doing, I reply "I am doing quite well" because I am.

Some persons, however, rather like the attention they get when they become ill, but after a while even they usually come to realize that it has gotten out of hand and they are not benefitting from it in any positive way.

I have observed that after a few months into the cancer challenge, many of the persons with whom you may have confided your condition, eventually tire of "checking on you" unless there has been some deterioration. They turn their attention back to their "business as usual" and you find that all you have left around you are a few of your real friends and family members. This can cause a sick person to feel very alone, almost like the feeling you get after the death of a very close relative when everyone goes back to their homes and their lives and you are left sitting at home, all alone, wondering "what just happened?"

There is definitely power in the prayers of others, but I believe that most persons who promise to "pray for you" never do so anyway and besides, if those persons who love you, dearly, pray for you, their prayers, along with your own faithful prayers and that of the elders in the church, are quite sufficient. God does not have to be reminded by hundreds of persons that you are in desperate need of His help. He already knows it before you were even diagnosed and He already knows how everything will turn out. Again, this is my personal opinion, but it works for me.

I need the attention of God and Him alone, I need His healing power. I need His assurance, His forgiveness, guidance, and mercy—because only God can heal me, no doctor, no treatment, no diet, nothing apart from God can do it, so that is who I rely on, solely. Rather than discussing my symptoms, disease, etc., with all those who would wish to know what is happening in my life, I use my time trying to develop my faith in God and endeavor to please Him and follow His commandments.

Although our faith can be strengthened over a period of time, we cannot have a part time faith, it must be a complete and total faith in His promises. It reminds me of how a child, at Christmas time, tells his parents and Santa Claus what he wants, then walks away, having complete faith that since he/she has been "good" that the parents/Santa will deliver on the request. He does not continue to write to Santa each week or remind the parents daily—the child has faith that he has made known his desire and that the parents/Santa will deliver. That is the kind of faith we must have.

We must strive for complete and unwavering faith, which we cannot allow anyone around us to shatter. Faith is our lifeline. We must believe it when God says that Heaven and Earth will pass away before any word from His mouth returns void.

Mind you, there are times when a child asks for something that is not in his own best interest, or in some instances, the parent has an even better gift in store for the child, so when Christmas comes, the parent ensures that the child, while not in every instance getting exactly what he wished for, the child gets what his loving parent knows **is best for him**. This is how it is with our God.

When God created the first family, He intended for them to have perfect health and a perfect life, but they chose to disobey him and thus we, through them, have to suffer the penalty for their disobedience. But Jesus came and died in order for us to receive forgiveness of our sins and to have hope for a better life. While it is not always perfect, through Him, it could, however, be much better than we expect it to be. In Psalms 23 we realize that there will be trials and tribulations, when it refers to our walking "through the valley of the shadow of death" but notice it does not say, being stuck there, rather it refers to **walking through** it, along it, out of it, IF we truly believe. We must get rid of fear as best we can.

Many times, in the Bible, Jesus told those persons around him to "FEAR NOT" because He was with them, just as He was with Daniel in the lions' den and with the three Hebrew young men in the fiery furnace. He promised never to leave us or forsake us, but we must first believe His word.

We must keep ourselves close to Him so that we can feel His presence when we are going through our trials. We must never give up, never! No matter the amount of pain, we must learn to push past the pain, knowing that He is always with us and when we do our best, He has promised to do the rest for us.

We must keep our eyes on Him, and do not be like Peter when he was walking on the water. When he took his eyes off Jesus, it was only then that he began to sink into the same water, on which a few moments before, he had been walking.

It is very sad but unfortunately quite true that, some persons, who maybe, even unconsciously, were very unhappy and unfulfilled prior to their diagnosis, use their disease to escape their sadness and feelings of being unloved and alone. Some cancer patients, prior to diagnosis, suffered for years with unfaithful spouses, abuse, others were disappointed in their children, some felt left out or trampled upon by life and those around them, and in these instances, many of them just allow themselves to sink further into the depths of despair and eventually welcome the escape that death affords.

To have any chance of survival, you must love and believe in God, you must love yourself and have an unwavering desire to live, a lust for life. To complete this life journey you have started, you must want to be a part of your family's future and have hopes and dreams for a future for yourself along with those you love.

Despite everything we have been led to believe, life during and after cancer can be wonderful and fulfilling, especially if you are a believer. You have the wonderful opportunity to encourage others through your own experiences. You have time, during this interruption of your normal routine, to rethink and reevaluate your life and dreams. Your life, no matter how long you get to live, can be much more focused and fuller than it was pre-cancer.

Life Lesson: In the words of Johnathan Winters:
If your ship does not come in, swim out to it!

Prior to the diagnosis, money and a secure financial future were my primary focus. My overwhelming concern was whether or not I was heading in the direction of financial security whereby I would be able to support myself at a standard I would be comfortable with after retirement. I had doubts whether or not I had adequately positioned myself, over years, to survive on my retirement benefits and the relatively small savings I would have had accumulated by my retirement date.

I was extremely comfortable with my health, I exercised regularly, I ate well, I was not overweight, my cholesterol was within limits. My blood pressure was just slightly elevated, but nothing to worry about, so I had no fears regarding my future health. I always had an annual physical and never neglected any health concerns I was faced with over the years.

My only concern, of consequence, was my ongoing lack of a good night's sleep. For some time now, I have had some challenges with the amount of sleep I get nightly. I usually wake up twice per night, either to use the bathroom or because of my snoring waking me up. Most times I go back to sleep easily, but it is still quite disruptive and some mornings I awake not entirely rested. This was not something that I was overly concerned with, especially as many of my friends expressed the same challenge. However, now faced with cancer, isn't it amazing how my focus has moved totally away from my finances, or sleep deprivation.

My spirituality, my health, my mortality, my future, my family, my independence, these are now my concerns. I remember when, just the night prior to my diagnosis, I was driving a long distance from home, late at night, and became a bit anxious about being alone on the streets. Now, that seems so insignificant when faced with possible "death from cancer." It is amazing what a difference a day makes.

Earlier on the same day of my diagnosis I had been worrying about my adult children, one of whom is presently out of work, but at this moment I cannot lend any energy to my children's lives or careers. She has assured me that they can survive on her husband's income for a few months. I will continue to pray that God helps her find employment and leave it there. I also worried about my grandchildren, the challenges they face in this world we live in, their futures. So often sleep evaded me due to my worrying about everyone and everything around me.

I am very aware that I was a compulsive worrier. I sometimes wonder if this excessive amount of worrying has taken a negative toll on my health and well-being because I do believe that worry and stress compromise our immune systems, among other things.

But, amazingly, in this short time, I have taken on a total change of focus and priority. I now fully recognize and accept that I can do nothing, on my own, to ensure my children's futures; I can do nothing from where I am in life to ensure my grand children's safety or future health or happiness. I cannot change anything by worrying and losing sleep.

On my own, I can do nothing of consequence about anything. I have now come to realize that I have no power over anything or anyone. God is in charge of everything: my life, my health, my future, my job, my finances, my children and my grandchildren. No matter what I eat, whether or not I undergo chemotherapy, whether or not my finances are in order, no matter what my diagnosis, ONLY God knows what the future will bring, only God and God alone. I must follow His lead for my life and try to hear his guidance in my spirit.

My whole thinking process has changed. My focus has turned completely around. I realize that this experience is all about me and my God. The God who created the universe and everything in it. He caused every individual grain of sand to be formed. He created every fingerprint on every human hand to be different and He looked down on His creation and declared "well done." Surely such a God can heal me IF that is His will and purpose for my life at this stage of my existence here on this earth. I accept that even if I am healed from this disease, no one lives forever, death is our reality.

I truly believe that everything that He allows to happen to us is for a reason, a very good reason. Most times we do not understand His reasoning, especially at first. But as time goes on and our faith and understanding of His word and His will increases in our life, so does our acceptance of His will for us, whether here on this earth or in the life beyond, because His will for us does not stop here on this earth. His will transcends this realm of our present existence and understanding.

This whole experience has humbled me tremendously. It has refocused my whole life. Prior to the diagnosis, I was totally engrossed in worrying about securing my financial future, now everything is different. The irony of it all is that now that I am faced with more medical expenses than I could ever have imagined, I am not in the least bit concerned about money or bills. Crazy, right?

Now, one surgery and about $35,000 in expenses later, my whole focus has completely changed. Thank God for my insurance coverage and His involvement in this whole experience. Shockingly, but obviously being led by the hand of God, my surgeon informed me that he will not charge me any of the co-pay. He will accept only what the insurance company pays him. Excluding upcoming radiation treatments, and medical oncologist's bills, my out-of-pocket is only $3,000 so far.

In this experience, it seems as if God is speaking directly to me saying, "I told you that if you believed, trusted and have complete faith in Me, I will take care of you." This is definitely the hand of God working for me and showing me His awesome power. There is no other explanation. My God is a good God, He is an awesome God and He never goes against His promise—that is, if we believe completely in Him and His power to protect, help and heal! It is all about Him.

Life lesson: I totally realize that all I need is Him, no one else—
just Him. When I require the involvement of a human being,
He will go ahead of me and arrange the perfect person to come into
my life to perform whatever I need done by them.

I realize that we have no power over what direction our lives will take from moment to moment. We have little control over what will happen in our lives, when or why or by whom or what. Isn't it amazing how persons can go to sleep at night, in an apparent healthy state, and never wake up the next morning? Acts of God, criminal acts, a massive stroke, heart attack or any other sudden death scenario, could wipe us out in an instant. In the vast majority of cases, we have no warning and even if we had some warning, we have no control over how the situation will eventually turn out. We could have good tenure on our job, with high performance ratings and by the end of the month, we may no longer have that "secure" job.

I was, obviously, completely oblivious to this possibility in my life—cancer? Now this faith and physical battle rages but, thankfully, God is in front of me.

Life lesson: We determine virtually nothing about our future.
Money cannot secure a long, healthy life any more than a long
life can ensure prosperity.

Being a human being, I do sometimes wonder,
How will this all turn out?
How long will it last?
What will happen along the way?
What will change most during the remainder of my life?

What, if anything, will be my constant burden?
What will be my greatest reward?
How will my emotional state be affected?
How will my life be improved?
What purpose does God have in mind for me?

What I do know for certain is that I desperately need God every moment of every day of my life, to lean on Him as well as His wisdom and guidance. Sometimes I feel like a child, a very scared little child who has fallen and hurt myself after having a false confidence in my ability to jump from one rock to another, and here it is now, I find myself clinging onto my Heavenly Father's arm for help and solace.

I refuse to let go of His hand. Whatever the future holds, I know He will always be there to help me through whatever I stumble over. I am holding on to His promise of forgiveness and healing, as I go through this tunnel, hopefully, towards "the light" of tomorrow.

As I continue to look within and ponder every aspect of my life, I find myself in a place of peace that I have not experienced in many years. I am actually sleeping a bit better, in fact, I have even had a dream or two recently. One scripture in the Bible has become the foundation for my peace and that is Jeremiah 29:11-14 which says," For I know the plans I have for you, says the Lord, plans for your welfare and not for harm, to give you a future with HOPE. Then, when you call upon Me, and come and pray to Me, I will hear you. When you search for Me, you will find Me; if you seek Me with all your heart, I will let you find Me, says the Lord."

These verses have become my compass. I have seen the lives of so many persons, from mega stars and mega millionaires, to the paupers along the street, cut down by cancer. The money, the prestige and the best doctors could not save the rich and powerful any more than "luck" could save the paupers. Only God knows our future. We must lean on Him and put our entire life in His hands.

I always remember when my favorite movie star, Michael Landon, was diagnosed with cancer. I remember that he immediately changed his eating habits, his whole lifestyle, he did everything "right." He had the absolute best doctors and medical facilities at his beck and call, and still he suffered and died. He, like the rest of us, had no control over anything; the same situation with my heroine, Farrah Fawcett. You just never know.

There are no guarantees that we control, but there is hope and faith that God will do what is His perfect will for our lives. The Bible says that He knew us and our future from the foundation of the earth. Long before we were formed in our mother's womb, He already knew how our life story would play out. It is said that life is a stage, if that is the case, then God is the writer/director/producer.

THE HEALING JOURNAL

I love to read but have realized that during this whole ordeal, so far, I have not been able to focus my mind on any substantial reading material. Even the latest work from my favorite author did not stir up in me a desire to pick up a book. I have been engrossed with research on everything cancer-related and now with the radiation treatments looming ahead of me, I decided I needed some diversion, some kind of light, uplifting reading.

I headed to a really well-stocked bookstore near my office, hoping to find something of interest, anything not cancer-related. My search proved futile so I began to look through the greeting cards section, which is also a favorite pastime of mine. I got a few good laughs from some of the cards, gathered a few to purchase and then strolled to the stationery section which housed gift boxes, bags and everything beautiful for gift-giving. I noticed an area that displayed photo albums, scrapbooks and journals. I picked up one of the journals and looked through it. It was a perfect size. It had some type of anecdote, famous saying or biblical quotation in a little corner, at the top of each page. As I held it, I noticed that it was bound in a soft, satin like, grass green fabric and it felt "right."

I have never kept a journal before. I never saw the value of it. I always thought that my private thoughts were meant to stay housed my own head and never to be placed on paper where anyone could possibly, eventually, read them. I live alone, but my friends as well as my children and grandchildren visit regularly. They are always in and out of my bedroom when they visit because that is where the only TV is located. A visible journal may jolt their natural curiosity to sneak a peek.

Despite my reservations regarding privacy, I just could not let go of it. I took it, without any specific intention for it, along with some cards, to the cashier, paid for everything and left the bookstore. It was weird in a way, but later that afternoon, I could not wait to get home to begin writing my thoughts and experiences of this "journey" in this new journal.

That night, after I ate, showered and settled in, I sat up wondering where to begin my recording and what particular aspect should I highlight. Needless to say, I did not know where to begin. I sat up almost half the night, thinking about what to write and eventually wrote nothing.

The following night, when I arrived home and while I was having my evening meal, the thought came to me that I was overthinking this whole thing. "Maybe I should just begin writing whatever comes into my mind," I thought to myself, and so I did.

Now, every night I grab the journal from my bedside table and jot down any experience, thought, question or success I have had that day or anything, for that matter, that I feel is worth transferring from my mind to the journal. A few days into recording my experiences, I realized that it was a real stress reliever. I looked forward to coming home and jotting down my thoughts and reactions to the things I did or heard (or said) during the day.

I intend to record this whole cancer experience. Journaling has become therapeutic. When I write, I become so engrossed in what I write, I lose all track of time (and pain) and just enter into another world completely.

I recommend anyone who is going through any experience, whether happiness, marriage, expecting a baby, sickness, doubt, confusion, divorce, job loss or anything that is filling your life or thought process, to begin journaling your every emotion, fear or success or any situation during the day that made an impact on you. Going back and reading what I had written is a wonderful encourager.

My "healing journal" as I began to call it, has also become my "gratitude journal." Each time I make an entry I realize how much there is to be grateful for and I make a note of everything that was positive and good in my day.

You may be thinking there is nothing positive in your life right now, everything seems to be spiraling downwards, but if you are reading this book, then it means that you can see, you can absorb the information and that you still have hope; and hope and faith are our biggest gifts in life when things are down and we feel lonely and depressed. There is hope. Just let your thoughts flow to your fingers and whatever comes to mind, just jot it down. Do not over think anything. It does not have to be grammatically correct or even make sense at the time, but it will eventually, when you look back at it. The more you write, the easier it gets. Try it. It is guaranteed to improve your mood and desire to press forward.

THE BLUE MAZDA

I remember the first car I ever bought. It was a blue Mazda. It was the most beautiful shade of blue, with leather seats and lots of leg room in front and back. Only once before had I ever noticed a blue Mazda on the streets. Immediately as I drove my "new" car on to the highway, blue Mazdas were everywhere. I noticed the same thing with my second and third cars as well. All of a sudden, whenever I got a particular car, duplicates surfaced everywhere.

So it is with cancer. As soon as I was diagnosed, all of a sudden it seemed as if there was an epidemic. Cancer is here, there and everywhere. So many people are battling this dreaded disease. It is all around us. Either someone you know is/was fighting it, or someone in their family or among their friends. Suddenly,

I realize how many television commercials are cancer-related, showing the different types of cancer, treatments and medical facilities that specialize in the treatment thereof.

It is amazing how we drift casually along life's highway oblivious to what is going on, simply because we are not experiencing it personally. It is very encouraging, however, to hear the wonderful survival stories, to learn so much about the disease, treatments, lifestyles, medical breakthroughs and most of all, the awesome miracles that occur daily. We are continually surrounded by miracles, and we live in hope that God has a miracle planned for us.

One such miracle story, I found out recently, concerns a young woman who works with me. Seven years ago she was diagnosed with Stage 4 stomach cancer. It had already spread to her liver, her ovaries and her colon by the time she was diagnosed correctly. Everyone around her doubted that she would ever recover. She is, however, a real believer, a very spiritual person who decided that whatever God's will was for her life, she would be content with it.

She decided, rather than mourn her condition and feel sorry for herself, she would continue looking to the future and continue her "normal" life to the best of her ability. She has always been grateful for everything and everyone in her life, maintained a positive attitude and always walk about with a big smile on her face.

She had major surgery, four series of chemotherapy treatments, a round of radiation and also underwent steroid treatments for some time as well. She was away from work for six months, lost all of her hair, but now one year later, she is doing very well, in remission and going on with her wonderful life. She is as happy as anyone can possibly be.

"How did this journey impact your life?" I queried. "What did you do differently?"

"Initially, as you can imagine, I was in total shock," she said. "I was young and afraid for my future, I wondered how I would deal with all the side effects, including the loss of my hair. I didn't know how it would impact my life and career. I prayed and decided to put the whole thing into God's hands and leave it there. I went on with my normal life, my adjusted eating habits and my regular routine," she said. "Although the doctors and most of my family thought I would not make it, I never doubted my full recovery, I just didn't!"

She changed nothing of consequence. When she returned to work, she was still bald, wore no wig, but held her head high, filled with pride and gratitude for her blessings. Can you believe it? It shows that God does not need any help from us when His plan is already in place to heal us.

So, I wait. Wait and hope and reflect. I reflect on all the time wasted in worrying rather than believing and thanking God for what I have, rather than what I want.

Note to Journal: Stop putting so many things off for later. Later may never come. In this, my "new" life, later will never be the same. Use every moment of every day to thank God for the miracle of life in fact, just waking up each morning is a miracle. Appreciate every day of life with family and friends. Waste no time. Pray constantly because everyone's days are numbered, sick or not.

DEATH IN THE FAMILY

Completely unexpectantly, my aunt called tonight to inform me that my 50-year-old favorite cousin, her son, was just diagnosed with late Stage 4 liver cancer. Everyone was shocked. No one suspected he was sick. In his late teens, early 20s, he was a heavy smoker and drinker, then a serious drug addict. But in his late 20s he completely transformed his life. We were all immensely proud of him. He was a great example to all the other cousins and the best example of how change is possible.

He worked hard and saved his money as well as helping his parents financially. Eventually he met a great girl and they married and raised three children over the years.

About 10 years ago, he was diagnosed with Hepatitis C and was placed on a strict diet and medicine regimen. Apparently after a few years of feeling healthy, he discontinued the treatments and resumed a not so healthy lifestyle. I do not know if this contributed to his present condition, but it did make me wonder.

I called and asked to speak to him but his wife said that he was very weak and unable to chat, but she will tell him that I called. She and I spoke for a while and then I tried to go off to sleep. As you can imagine, sleep completely evaded me. I thought of how close we were before his "druggie" days and how we resumed our relationship after his turnaround and how much sound advice he gave me over the years. He was always the life of the party.

After we both married, had careers and children of our own, except for the occasional large family reunions, we drifted a bit apart. However, when my husband died, he pitched in and was a great help with my children, especially my son, who needed a father image in his life. After my children were grown, I moved to Central Florida, after a job offer but he and my children remained in close contact.

Consumed with my own health battle, I had not spoken to him in a few months and assumed all was well with him. He and my children live nearby and remain quite close, so I will let them know tomorrow so they can visit him.

The phone jolted me awake the next morning at 5:45 and immediately I knew it was bad news. During the night his condition deteriorated rapidly and he had to be transported, by ambulance, to the hospital. He died a few hours later. Long after I hung up the phone from his oldest son, I just stared at it. I felt as if everything had drained from my body. I would have collapsed had I not been sitting on the edge of my bed.

What had just happened? He could not be dead. He seemed so healthy in June at his 50th birthday party. How long was he aware of the cancer? Did he just find out this week? Surely not! He must have suffered some really debilitating pain. Did he share his condition with his wife? I did not think to ask her about that when we spoke last night. A million unanswered questions filled my brain, the biggest one now being, how do I tell my children what just happened overnight? How will they receive the news? Will this news make them more concerned for my struggle with this dreaded disease?

I sat completely still for about half an hour, my head overwhelmed with thoughts and regrets, especially for being so concerned for myself that I did not call him recently. How painful he must have been? How afraid? Did he share with his immediate family, and if not, how lonely he must have been? I kept thinking of how supportive he was when my husband died.

When I finally pulled myself together, I picked up the phone and called my oldest daughter. She had to pass the phone over to her husband, she was so overcome with grief. My cousin was like her "other dad." She said that she had spoken to him within the past few weeks and he said that he was fine. How could this happen? To avoid putting me through this again, she said that she would call her siblings before she went over to his home to be with his wife and family. I then called my aunt, who was inconsolable and finally his wife who I had hoped to comfort until my daughter arrived. She was in such a state of shock that the conversation was short. She was in no condition to chat.

The funeral was on the weekend and I drove up for it. I stayed at my younger daughter's home and was not prepared for the grief and pain she and the grandchildren were undergoing. It made me wonder what would happen if I were to die in the near future from this cancer. It blew my mind. Despite every effort to control myself, I broke down. By the time my older daughter and my son came by, I had to take a couple aspirin to cope. My head was hurting and my cancer struggle became very real. All the questions I had avoided, now filled my head; I even started to picture my own funeral. Of course, I did not wish my family to realize what I was going through, so I put on a brave face and busied myself with preparing a meal for the after-funeral family dinner.

I was numb during the funeral, during the dinner afterwards and for the drive home the following afternoon, which I did despite my family's threats to take away my keys for another day or two, but I was scheduled to begin the radiation treatments on Monday so I had to leave the Sunday afternoon. All I could think about was, what if this was my death and funeral, how would my family cope? I realized I was not only mourning for my cousin, but for myself as well. Hopefully, the long drive home would be a perfect distraction from my thoughts.

I played a few genres of music during the three-hour drive home. I realized that I had to get my affairs in order the following week, just in case. I was in a state of depression for at least another two weeks. I had to force myself to "turn my eyes toward Jesus" and begin to replace sadness and doom with faith and hope. It took much discipline and determination, but life must go on, so rather than moping about, I intentionally returned to my routine and thanked God for the gift of each new day.

RADIATION TREATMENTS

It is now two months post-surgery. Today, I am scheduled to meet with the doctor at the radiation center for the initial radiation consultation, prior to the beginning of the treatments. After the usual health questions and reviewing the information from the radiation oncologist, he explained the procedure. I will come in five days per week, from 12:15 p.m. to 12:45 p.m. for six weeks and the technicians will administer the pre-determined amount of radiation to the affected area.

He said that I would be "tattooed" around the area that will receive the radiation prior to the commencement of the therapy, because each patient's radiation therapy is different and very specific to each individual case. The area must be tattooed to ensure there is no mix up of where the treatment is to be administered. As well, my picture must be taken and attached to my file to act as daily confirmation that the correct procedure and dosage is being administered to the correct patient.

He warned that the surgical scar along the breast area (from the nipple down to about two inches under the breast), may be impacted by the effects of the radiation. He advised that the treatments may cause a widening of the scar. He said that there will be some itching in the area being treated, and suggested that I liberally apply cornstarch as needed. He suggested that I be careful with the skin of the breast, never to "rub" it hard, just very gently wash the area with my hands using very mild soap. He said, "treat the area as you would the skin of a newborn baby."

He further stated that the skin area that is being radiated will turn a darker color "like a dark suntan." He warned that, in some cases, the after-effects do not manifest themselves until after the treatment period is over. Finally, he gave me some written information to review, after which a nurse came in and whisked me away to the changing room, a room with which I was to become familiar over the next six weeks.

I was instructed to remove all clothing, above my waist, along with my glasses and any jewelry, even my watch as my hand had to be lifted above my head to perform the radiation process. I then had to put on the, now all too familiar, paper gown with a front opening and then wait my turn to go into the "chamber." I was surprised how busy the center was.

I think the radiation chamber was built and equipped so that no radiation would escape. It had the appearance of a large vault with a specially designed door.

When I was escorted into the chamber I was instructed to lie on my back. They turned my head to the right side, while my left arm was placed on a bracket, of sorts, while I held on to a bar, above my head. This posture allowed them to have full access to my left breast and the area underneath as well as under my armpit, the area from where the lymph nodes had been removed. I was very nervous during the tattooing and first treatment, particularly after being told about all the possible side/after-effects

Having to remain "very still" in this position, caused my arm and shoulder to become very tense and tired. The first day's procedure took an hour as they had to take pictures, perform the tattoo and x-rays prior to the official commencement of the treatment. They do this in order to have on file, a "before" record. Each Wednesday they would be taking pictures and x-rays to compare with the original pictures, which would allow them to gauge my progress.

The technicians were very warm and caring. They were both young and eager to perform at their best. One was originally from South Africa and the other hailed from New York. They were quite patient and understanding when I complained of how difficult it was to hold steady in the position for the half hour treatment. They continually encouraged me to relax and assured me that as the treatments progressed, the process would be much less uncomfortable. They asked that I make a note of any concerns I may have, as I would be seeing the chief radiologist once per week, on Wednesdays, after the regular treatment.

By the end of the first week, I had experienced no side effects and the procedure became more bearable as I learned to relax. It was at the end of the second week that I noticed that the scar, under the breast, appeared to have widened a bit. I continued to care for the area very carefully and used the corn starch as instructed.

When I returned to work after the surgery, I realized that I was still unable to perform my household chores without discomfort, so I hired the services of a Maid to come in on Saturdays to assist with the housekeeping, some laundry and lifting my grocery bags upstairs. I am indebted to my best friend for her tremendous assistance for a month, but I realized I needed ongoing help after I returned to work. Although this was absolutely not in my budget, it was necessary. I will keep her until I feel comfortable to do everything on my own. I have no desire to do anything to compromise my healing.

I live alone and as the procedure continued, I realized that the Maid and I may have a longer relationship than I had originally anticipated. This ongoing new expenditure is putting a big dent into my finances, but it is absolutely necessary to my ongoing healing and welfare. I hope that after a few more weeks, I can revert to cleaning my home myself. I will test myself every couple weeks to see how much I can do around the condo. My children take turns visiting me twice monthly, are happy that I have help around the house as well as the fact that, until now, the radiation treatments are bearable.

In the third week of radiation the skin covering the scar began to separate and the under layer of the skin became exposed. It reminded me of when a boil bursts and the under layer of skin is exposed. The very gradual swelling of the breast/chest area caused by the radiation treatment, forced the skin to stretch apart. The scar gradually reddened and continued to widen.

What was a perfectly stitched surgical scar, now took on the shape of an upside-down tornado—with the top thereof being where the chest joined the bottom of breast and gradually narrowing as it got closer to the nipple. It is becoming increasingly uncomfortable when the skin of the breast touches the skin of my chest. I hope no rash or further abrasion happens, as this could negatively impact the healing process. It takes quite a bit of effort and patience to ensure the area stays dry.

Octobers are still quite warm and humid here, so before I go outdoors, I apply plenty of corn starch to avoid sweat from affecting the scarred area. At nights I sleep topless, on my back for as long as I can, to ensure the area stays dry. I have never intentionally slept on my back before and it is taking quite a lot of getting used to. After a few sleepless nights it became a bit more bearable. Never really comfortable, but bearable. Sleeping on my back causes me to snore. So, when I would finally fall off to sleep, my snoring and dry mouth would choke/jolt me awake, OMG! I have to keep a glass of water on the nightstand to quench my parched mouth. This is exceedingly difficult and I am losing a lot of sleep.

During one of the weekly visits to the chief radiologist, he asked, "Have you started to feel more tired? This is a common side effect." I smiled, shook my head and thought before I responded. "Yes," I said. But in my mind, I said to myself, "Yes, I am more tired, and yes, I feel like hell. I have a scar that is causing me excruciating pain and discomfort, in addition I am trying to adjust to sleeping on my back."

All of my life I have slept on my left side and now I can no longer sleep on my left side because the "bones may become slightly more brittle due to the radiation." So, lying on my back or my right side are my only options. When I lay on the right side, the left breast hangs over and feels like the skin is pulling apart, so that became a non-option. As if that were not enough, I am faced with, what I consider, inflated medical bills from this procedure and he asks me if I am tired? "Yes," I quietly replied, "I am more tired" (but unlike what he was referring to, I am now becoming weary of this whole situation, the side effects and the loss of energy. I am unable to distinguish if it is specifically the radiation treatments or the whole ordeal that is causing me to feel completely exhausted.

The fourth week brought on a new challenge: shooting pains in the breast area. They were "off and on" so, in the beginning, I did not take any pain medication. They came on quite suddenly and were sharp. My body would jerk impulsively when they came. After a couple of minutes, they would disappear. This new side effect, continued all day, off and on for several weeks afterwards. Sometimes, at nights, if the pains were particularly sharp that day, I would take pain medication or a sleeping pill to get some relief overnight. This was particularly disconcerting at work, because I did not wish anyone to notice. I was thankful my cubicle is at the rear of the larger room.

Today the doctor whose clinic mis-read my mammogram and under-evaluated the level of cancer in the breast/lymph nodes prior to the surgery, called me. Although, in my heart, I felt she was to "blame" for the cancer reaching Stage 2, my faith in God's purpose for my life has now overshadowed the two doctors' mistakes, but my human self was not yet ready to speak to her. Maybe in time, but not yet. I was happy I was not at home and the call went to my answering machine.

Also, during the same week, a category 2 hurricane threatened the lower and upper east coast of the United States. I had to rush out quite early, before work, and purchase a pane of glass for my kitchen window. I installed it that evening. Something so simple, I put off for so long. As I usually do, I had the maintenance crew at my complex, install the shutters over the windows and sliding glass door. Although I also went grocery shopping, I did not have to purchase many items, because I had been gradually stocking up from the beginning of the summer. I purchased batteries, water and fruits as well as items to replenish my first aid kit.

The radiation center called early on the morning of the storm's pending approach and asked me to come in right away as they were closing at 11:00 a.m. due to the storm's passage. I immediately dropped everything and went in. Our office, like most other businesses, closed at 12pm. The following day we felt the biggest impact of the storm and everything remained closed, including the radiation center. I regarded the break with mixed feelings although it gave the breast area some time to rest a bit.

Although the Hurricane did not come inland, it passed not too far offshore and we experienced Tropical Storm force winds and heavy rains. My roof sounded as if it was about to lift off. As long as we had phone service, me and my children were checking on each other. Thankfully, we all fared well. Our city remained closed for two days afterwards because of downed trees, power lines and flooded streets. She did not directly hit us, but Hurricane Sandy wreaked havoc along the northern East Coast of the U.S. Many buildings were either destroyed or badly damaged and the area did not recover for quite a while. There was loss of life and billions of dollars of damage.

I could not help wondering what happened to the radiation patients in those areas where treatments were interrupted for much longer periods of time due to the damage from the storm. I only missed three treatments which will push back my treatment schedule a bit.

I hate the "sticking" pains, they just show up out of nowhere and choose any random spot on the breast area to attack. The radiologist advises these are "normal" and to be expected, but these pains could have the courtesy to call first or give me a bit of notice prior to their arrival. Just as I am writing about it, at this very moment, "Mr. Sticky Pain" decides to pop his ugly head in. Well, fella, I am going to ignore you.

Mind over matter, sometimes. I am amazed at how, after ignoring the pain for a while, it usually ceases or at least, diminishes and after a time, you realize it is gone. This is not the case with seriously intense pain, of course, and sometimes it is impossible to ignore, but, other times, you have the choice of either allowing it to "take over" or doing your best to ignore it. I choose to ignore it whenever possible. Whenever it persists for any noticeable period of time, I take something for it, but 99 percent of the time, it goes away after I turn my attention to my daily routine.

In the normal course, by the middle of November, I would have been busy planning out my Christmas card list in order to dispatch them just after Thanksgiving. I would have already begun to organize my Christmas gift shopping list and most likely I would have already been planning a small party at my home, for some of my close friends as well as my annual family Christmas dinner bash. Not this year! My only focus is completing the radiation treatments (end date scheduled for just after Thanksgiving) and try to begin gradually reducing these escalating medical bills, which, even with insurance are quite steep.

Thank God my radiation oncologist promises, if at all possible, to try to negotiate with the radiation/cancer center to write off a portion of the co-pay for me. This will help tremendously.

When I get home nowadays, rather than sitting around and planning for Christmas, it takes all my remaining energy to complete the second half of the twice daily care of the breast. During my shower I, very gently, hand lather the breast with a mild soap, then pour a container of water over the area (the shower stream is too harsh for the breast at this time) then delicately pat the area completely dry.

From the date of the surgery until about a week or two into the radiation sessions, I had lost about seven pounds, but I now find myself '*stress-eating*' and have put the weight back on. I surely have no extra cash to purchase new clothes, so note to self, I must stop eating so many extra carbs. I wonder if I am supposed to be doing any light exercises at this time. I have discontinued my exercise regimen because with every move I make, I feel it in and under my left breast so I cannot rely on that option, at this time, to lose weight.

I am at the end of the fourth week and the surgical scar has widened yet a bit more and the "sore" is now larger as well. The breast also hurts more intensely. I am very meticulous in attending to its care, ensuring that I only use soap with no perfumes or dyes or anything that is less than 100 percent pure. I wear only very loose cotton undergarments over the breast area. I keep it clean and dry at all times, which requires an hourly bathroom run while at work. I keep cornstarch in my handbag which I apply as well. The swelling is now more obvious. The area is not as "sunburned" as I had been led to expect, only the under-arm lymph node area, which is now quite dark and hair is no longer growing in the left armpit.

So happy to be beginning the fifth week. The skin under the breast/chest area has now begun to take on the appearance of burned skin. It has begun to fold over itself and some ridges are appearing. I had been instructed at the beginning of the treatments, not to use any oils, lotions, creams or ointments of any sort on the area, only cornstarch to keep it dry, but this now appears more serious and I will speak with the doctor about it.

I went to see my radiation oncologist today and she advised "Great news, I was successful in arranging some financial assistance for you. The center has agreed to waive the radiation co-payments effective the third week of treatments." "Thank you, thank you, thank you," I squealed. I was so happy and overcome with gratitude I barely heard anything she said afterwards, but I do remember her suggesting that I use the gel of the Aloe plant on the affected area, and some olive oil after I shower at night. The oil will make the skin more pliable and should prevent further widening of the scar and the Aloe should heal the skin.

Thank goodness, the olive oil did ease the tightness of the skin but the healing was still very slow. I am very thankful that I am not yet suffering from the intense itching that so many experience after radiation treatments. Maybe it is because I have been smothering the entire area with cornstarch. The olive oil is doing a great job in lubricating the skin and keeping it pliable.

We all must take some personal responsibility for our individual care. There is always so much more to be learned apart from what our doctors say. I think they rely on our being willing/able to inform ourselves as much as possible about our condition and what to expect. There are books, magazines, support groups, and various lectures at medical facilities that are available for our use.

I read as much as possible about the care of the breast, diet, radiation, exercise of the arm area and was reminded that a great deal of an individual's recovery depends on his/her emotional stability, attitude and expectations of how your particular case will turn out in the end. I once heard a doctor say, "Most persons who believe they will die from cancer, usually do and most persons who have every faith and hope to survive, usually do, or at least much longer than even the doctors expected."

It seems most survivors program their minds with positive and healing thoughts. They are prepared to take their share of the responsibility for research and care, truly believing that they will get through and past this challenge.

The widening scar where my breast connects to my chest is now growing scar tissue and is feeling more uncomfortable with each passing day. It has now become difficult to wear close fitting camisoles (I wear sports tops and camisoles to make sure my breasts do not "jiggle about," especially the left one, because of my not being able to wear a bra). The shooting pains in the breast area are now becoming much sharper.

I see the radiation doctor each Wednesday (for no more than 5 mins.) As usual, he asks how I am feeling and although I tell him of the increasing pains, he assures me that everything is going as expected. In fact he, along with the radiation technologists, complimented me on how healthy and resilient my skin was, and if I recall correctly, I actually believe the word "remarkable" was used, but it is very difficult to feel remarkable when the scar, itself, seems so damaged and I continue to experience constant shooting pains. To appease myself, after a while, I began to call them "healing pains" and that took the edge off a bit, a very tiny bit. I am pleased with myself that over the years, I paid so much attention to skin care, as it seems to now be paying off, according to the doctors, anyway.

The skin is now quite dark and parched under the breast area and I remain concerned about the sore along the scar area. I was instructed to continue use of the aloe gel and olive oil, but one day I forgot to use the aloe and I noticed that the sore dried up significantly more than when I used it, so I made a decision to only use the olive oil, for a while, anyway.

It worked! After a few days the skin became more pliable and the sore showed definite signs of healing. I cannot explain why the area healed more rapidly without the aloe gel; it could have been a coincidence of timing or maybe the use of the olive oil alone, at that stage. Whatever it was, it worked and I am ecstatic.

During the fifth week the scar at the bottom of my armpit, from the lymph node surgery, began to "sing" a bit louder. This has never posed much of a problem before. All of a sudden, it began to be even more easily irritated by clothing and sometimes, just for the heck of it, it would really hurt. The skin around the scar began to feel very tight, almost as if it would tear apart if I raised my arm up too high. I decided to cover that area with the olive oil as well.

As you can imagine, all of my under garments, undershirts, camisoles, everything, are all covered with oil stains. What the heck, they are the trophies of this war.

Some nights the pain in my armpit forces me to take painkillers which, thankfully, allow me to drift off to sleep. I had to purchase some wider armed underwear and blouses to avoid further irritation of the underarm area.

Up to this point, for the most part, I had been very upbeat and my spirits high. My faith has never wavered because I fortify myself with God's word, and daily experience His blessings. On this day, however, a Saturday morning, I awoke with a heavy heart. A sense of loneliness enveloped me. I suspected these feelings were inevitable somewhere along this journey. Well, here they are now.

As I opened my eyes this morning, there it was. My human nature took ownership of my thoughts. Mind you, it was a beautiful sunny morning in late November, about 73 degrees outside, with a nice breeze blowing off the coast. I looked outside my upstairs bedroom window and what was normally a feeling of awe as the sun's rays slowly peeped over the trees and through the blinds, had now become just an empty feeling. Not sadness, but just a lack of any particular emotion. An emptiness.

Early mornings are my favorite time of the day, but not today, there was just apathy. I had no appreciation for the beautiful golden and peach-colored rays as the sun rose higher and higher over the trees and the other buildings outside my window. The colors of the sunrise (and sunset) change daily and even the direction of the sun changes as the seasons change and observing those periods are my favorite pastimes, because I love nature.

I always look forward to walking to the beach and staring at the sea as the tides rise and fall and watch the waves, sometimes angrily, splash over the rocks and at other times, just gracefully slither over them. I love to see it all, but not today.

I lay there asking myself "What could possibly have changed so drastically overnight." One thought kept popping up in my brain—desertion! I suddenly realized that two of the eight persons in whom I had confided my illness, had not called me in weeks to check on me or my progress. It was hard to believe that one quarter of my closest friends in whom I had confided, had deserted me.

Excluding family, the health care professionals, my boss and the human resources manager, I have only told eight persons about my challenge, and to think that two of them have backed away from dealing with it, was a total shock to me. It was actually physically painful. I trusted these few persons above everyone else who I called "friends" and I have many friends, but now, not a word, call or even a text/e-mail from two of the eight persons I esteemed to be my closest friends.

The more I thought about it, the more I came to realize that many people are unable to handle such weighty news or the responsibility it brings. They immediately become selfish and decide they are "unable to deal with it." I guess they feel that cancer brings with it, impending death and they decide to protect themselves from that painful thought.

They obviously decided to ignore the whole situation and pretend it never happened. I imagine they decided to hide out until, either I officially "survived," or died, only in this way could they go on with their lives. Looking back now, I realize that my decision to include them in this very important period of my life, was a matter of poor judgment on my behalf. I should have known better. This is just one of the painful lessons you learn along life's highway. Many people are unable to deal effectively with stress. "Fair-weather friends" is what they were referred to when I was a child. I wonder if they were waiting for me to contact/call them and give them progress reports, and I would have, had they shown even the slightest bit of concern.

You realize that only time and life determines who your real friends are. I never realized the extent of their selfishness. We all have different characters and different responses to "bad" news. Some people are so "hollow" they have no problem hearing about the misfortunes of others, because it makes them feel better about themselves, but cannot deal with anything that is negative that involves those close to them. I thank God for my real, through it all, friends who love and care, despite their own personal feelings, through the good times and the bad.

Lesson learned: Keep your eyes focused on Jesus and His promises and rid yourself of the expectations of others.

After identifying the "feeling" I woke up with, and dealing with it, I enjoyed the remainder of the day and had a great night's sleep.

The following day I decided to totally enjoy the sunset. I tossed my lonely and sad feelings of yesterday to the wind, so they can disappear over the horizon along with the setting sun. The bottom line: Do I believe God or not? As I sit here watching the sun and my depression of yesterday, sink over the horizon, I decided against scolding myself for slipping backwards for just a moment, but rather realize that I am human. Sometimes when we carry heavy loads, we begin to feel flustered and frazzled and become upset with ourselves and our lot in life.

It is during these times we have to fight, not to let the swirl of events going on all around us, to get into us. In these instances, I encourage myself and lean on God's help to slow down my thoughts and quiet my mind. This requires a very deliberate effort because, at times, it is easier to worry than to pray but prayer and meditation on His word will be the crane that lifts us up.

After sitting a while on the bench overlooking the shore, I wondered why I had become so worried because, now, watching the beautiful, big sun ball sink over the horizon, the problems and worries of the past few days/weeks seem strangely dim and distant. Sitting here, I can only vaguely remember why I became so worried. Many people nowadays are drowning in fear, doubt, lack of faith, restlessness, despair and loneliness. I refuse to be one of them.

I refuse to allow wayward friends to rob me of my happiness. Each day I will keep myself encouraged by what Jesus said in John 14:27, "Peace I leave with you, My peace I give to you. I do not give to you as the world gives. Do not let your hearts be troubled and do not let them be afraid." I will continually remind myself of this promise.

We must keep focused on Him! As soon as we allow our anxieties and cares to come between us and God, then problems happen, every time. I am now determined to keep my eyes, ears and mind totally focused on His love, His promises and His perfect will for my life.

Lesson to self: I will not let anyone or any circumstance come between me and my God.

This experience has taught me that with an army of two (God and I) I am stronger than all my friends and family members combined. I always lean on the words of one of my favorite spiritual songs when I am overwhelmed. It is written by Helen Howarth Lemmel and it reminds me to "Turn Your Eyes upon Jesus, look full in His glorious face, and the things of earth, will grow strangely dim, in the light of His glory and grace" God has promised me that He will never leave me or forsake me. Yesterday is over and I am done with it.

Today begins the sixth and final week of radiation treatments. This week's treatments are called the "Boost." The doctor said, "The boost is an amplified version of the doses given during the past five weeks. This week's treatments will concentrate on a very specific area of the breast and underarm, the area where the tumors were discovered in the breast and lymph nodes." Probably this week's treatments will ensure they have "burned" away all possible cancer cells around the previously affected area. So far, the treatments this final week feel no different from all the other treatments. What a blessing!

Today is the final day of the "boost." I have just received the last "burn" the super-duper one. Praise the Lord it is finished! At this stage, the area under my armpits has the look of crispy, burned bacon or maybe even lumps of lava left from a volcano and the top area of the breast is now darkening rapidly, as predicted. Also, the skin around the scar, under the breast, seems to be overlapping.

Thankfully, the sore that had begun to grow along the line of the scar at the bottom of the breast, seems to be healing a bit. The area around the scar, however, is now covered with dark pigments, almost like tiny polka dots on a crushed piece of fabric.

My sad looking left nipple, which is obviously a victim of this war, now points downward permanently due to the skin having been pulled down during the stitching of the breast during the lumpectomy surgery. My poor "little girl" (which is now what I call my left breast) not only looks downtrodden and sad, but she is very painful. Whenever I touch it by mistake, it is as if someone took a knife and stabbed me.

I can't believe it! Today, the long-dreaded itching has begun. The "boost" obviously caused the breast area to swell, again. It feels as if the skin is about to tear apart and it itches intensely. I just want to grab the breast and rub it with a piece of sandpaper to make the itching go away, but instead, I will increase both the cornstarch in the day and the olive oil at nights after my shower.

My co-workers would be shocked if they had any idea the suffering I am enduring.

Lesson: You have NO idea what persons, even those sitting near to you, are going through. Be kind, always.

Cancer is an awful enemy, so the fight to kill it entails a strategic battle plan on the part of the victim. After the final super-duper boost, I had to "consult" with the radiation doctor. So here I am, again, in my paper gown, sitting in his office. I still marvel at the fact that there are still three doctors dealing with me during the same period for the same disease. After the examination, he assures me that everything went very well and that he is pleased with the progress.

As I leave his office, and after thanking his wonderful team of radiation technicians and the pleasant office staff, I then drove directly to the radiation oncologist's office. She was also taking weekly pictures. She takes out the pictures she snapped over the past weeks and compares them to how the area looks today and advises that she, also, is pleased with the progress. "There will be some pain and discomfort for a while still but that is not unusual." I remember her telling me this at the beginning of the treatments.

She asked that I return for a follow-up visit in six weeks. She, again, strongly suggested that in the meantime, I see a medical oncologist to discuss chemotherapy options. I promised her I would. I maintain, however, that I refuse to BURN and then POISON my body. One is enough for me. I agreed to radiation but I will not add to the destruction by poisoning it as well. I will now immerse myself in natural healing methods that, I personally believe, have virtually all the benefits of chemotherapy but none of the poisoning and other damaging effects.

I have seen too many of my friends suffer and then die after not being able to recover from side effects of the damaging effects of chemotherapy. Their already ailing bodies could not withstand the side effects and they just deteriorated further and suffered longer. Some of my friends who survived the chemotherapy, are now, years later, experiencing various sorts of negative post side effects.

One is presently suffering from "drug resistance" due, she says, to her multiple chemotherapy treatments more than ten years ago. She now has to take two shots per week for five weeks to, hopefully, undo some of the effects of chemotherapy, so that she can take medicine prescribed for another ailment.

In the case of those who died, obviously the chemotherapy did not "heal" them. In my opinion, it only lengthened and intensified their suffering and cost them every penny they had. So, no matter how much urging my doctors give, I will not submit to chemotherapy treatments. I have placed my life in the hands of Jesus and will do everything in my power to free my mind of stress, worry and doubt, as He has commanded. I will cleanse my body from all impurities, as best I can, and refill it with natural, healing foods. The rest is up to Him, not man, who cannot even heal himself. As promised, however, I will make an appointment to see the medical oncologist.

I contacted my surgeon and advised him that the radiation treatments were now over and like my radiation oncologist, he too, again, suggested that I see the medical oncologist. I promised to. My surgeon, while completely understanding and accepting of my personal views on chemotherapy, was pleased with my decision.

AM I WINNING THIS BATTLE?

To answer this question, I will have to revert to my faith in God and my inherent warrior spirit. I have total faith in God's promises to forgive my sins and heal my diseases, according to His will and purpose for my life. I continue to read and lean on His promises in Psalm 91 and especially verses 14–16 which says: "Those who love me, I will deliver; I will protect those who know my name. When they call to me, I will answer them. I will be with them in trouble. I will rescue them and honor them. With long life I will satisfy them and show them my salvation."

Another portion of the Psalms, Chapter 103, verses 2–5 says "God forgives our sins, He heals our diseases, He redeems us from life's pitfalls and crowns us with His steadfast love and mercy, He satisfies us with good as long as we live, so that our youth is renewed like the eagle's." These are my go-to verses whenever I feel overwhelmed. They give me hope to press on.

Even after the passing of my husband, when I was steeped in doubt and fear, and second-guessed God, He was faithful and took perfect care of me and my children. Now that I am older and more involved with real life, I can see how He brought me through so many turbulent situations when I did not even acknowledge Him or thank Him enough. I realize that my life, my healing and my future is not dependent, specifically on what I eat, if I exercise, how I think or what I chant, etc. it is all up to Him and His will and purpose for my life. I am blessed that He has chosen me to go through this test to prove that He is still on the Throne. He is still the Great Physician and able, if it is His will, to heal me completely.

I want my life to be a full testimony to His awesomeness and the fact that He is still in the Healing business. My part in this relationship is to honor Him, obey His word, and lean on His promises. Just as a young child has complete faith and total belief in a parent's promises, we must have that same type of unequivocal faith that He will do as He has promised in His word.

I do believe, however, that we must take the best care of our bodies (which the Bible refers to as the "temple"). We must stay active and exercise discipline in our lives; this includes not overeating or becoming drunkards. We must guard our hearts, our minds and our mouths and we must pray and thank God for his faithfulness daily.

We must rid our hearts and minds of all unforgiveness, anger, bitterness and jealousy, as these emotions eat away at our soul/body. It is a fact that stress related diseases are rampant in today's world. We must learn to cry out to God and ask Him to help us with whatever is causing us emotional pain and suffering because our damaged emotions stunt our ability to heal from diseases.

> **Life lesson:** No one is immortal! Death is coming to everyone.
> We have no idea exactly when our name will be called, so stay
> focused on today, it has so much to offer. Live life to the max,
> and use each hour of every day to praise Him.

In order to cleanse our hearts and minds of all unrighteousness, we must purge our beings of everything detrimental to our spiritual and physical healing. Remember that God is good all the time, and He responds to our cry for help in His time. We must realize that His time is not always our time and while we are waiting for Him, we should stay positive and fill our lives with deeds of goodness and gratitude. This is the time for us to share with others, a portion of what has been gifted to us. Rather than sit around and worry, wonder and whine, why not go out and be an encouragement to others less fortunate than we are?

We must ensure the words we speak are reflective of what is true and pure and beneficial to us as well as others. The world is filled with persons in need of what we take for granted each day. Our gifts can be financial, a prayer, a word of encouragement, or a cake on someone's birthday. Many persons would appreciate an outfit you have outgrown, a bowl of soup, a jacket or sweater to someone in a Retirement home, a chocolate bar, a shoulder to lean on when someone needs to vent, a bottle of perfume that you are no longer attached to, anything that you can share.

I love to send greeting cards to persons with whom I have not communicated for a while, just to say "Hello." Sometimes when I go through my old pictures, I find extras. I then place them in a card and send them to the persons pictured therein and always, always, I get a call of thanks, with the recipient being so grateful and uplifted by the "gift."

Giving takes my mind off myself and my issues and fills me with a good feeling. I actually believe that healing is magnified when we take our minds off ourselves and concentrate on the needs of others. Last month, I bought a new pot set and donated my existing set to a senior home near me. They were so happy, they asked me to stay for dinner. I have now "adopted" some of the residents there.

Friend, this is the time to get busy, not to coil up in self-pity and doubt. After wiping away your tears, go and wipe away the tears of other persons who are going through similar or maybe different life challenges.

An old adage goes, "God helps those who help themselves" so help yourself by helping others. I am blessed that He has chosen me to go through this test to prove to myself, my family and friends that He is still on the throne, He is still in charge and more specifically to this moment in my life, He is still in the healing business.

He has promised me that he will never leave me or forsake me and that His promises will not return to Him void. He promises that Heaven and Earth will pass away before one word uttered from His mouth returns void. I constantly remind myself that God says that this battle is not mine, it is His own, so I leave the fighting to Him. I cannot wait to get well enough to share my journey with all my friends and church friends, but for now, I need this healing time to myself.

Yes, I believe with all my heart that my God is winning this battle waged against me by the evil one. If you are a believer in the God above, make it a habit to meditate on His word daily. Constantly repeat His promises to us. Sing songs of praise to continually uplift yourself. Allow God's word to be your main medicine. We get sick for many different reasons, sometimes it can even be from sin, so first of all, confess your sins and ask for His forgiveness.

The world is full of contaminants, toxic waste, viruses, germs, bad lifestyle habits, bad food and bad drinks. There are also what are referred to as generational diseases, i.e. diabetes, high-blood pressure, addictions, heart disease and the like. We must pray and work against these challenges in our lives. In these instances, from early on, we must do our part in changing our lifestyles and eating habits to invest in the best health possible despite what our parents or other family members may suffer from. God is the Great Physician and healing comes through Him alone, but as He instructs us in His word, we must be disciplined in our personal habits.

Obey God, maintain a positive outlook on life, trust in Him. Believe that the universe (life) is unfolding as it should. We must eat right, exercise, endeavor to keep stress at a minimum. We must let go of anger and bitterness. Allow sickness and diseases to become a bridge to a better spiritual life for yourself. Grow your relationship with God. Let your challenges become steppingstones to a closer relationship with Him. Honor Him and His great works in your life. Share the good news.

We must learn how to be happy and hopeful in the midst of adversity. We must use our experience as a tool to comfort others through our example of strength, faith and belief that whatever happens, God is still in charge and He will help us through, once we put all of our trust in Him. The more we desire healing and believe that God can heal us or deliver us through our sickness, the better our life will become. He knows what is best for us and if we agree with His word and believe in His perfect will for our lives, then we are already on the road to success. We must remind ourselves that this earthly life is only a portion of our total experience. He has promised us eternal life with Him.

The series of radiation treatments are now behind me and, thankfully, despite the burning, swelling, skin eruptions, sharp pains and itching during the treatment period, the doctors have said that everything went very well. While I am reminded that the worst of the side effects may happen now after the series of treatments are completed, at least there will be no surprises, so hopefully I will bear it without too much anxiety.

It is now two weeks since the end of the treatments and despite the fact that I am still experiencing the skin darkening and the scar under the breast has begun to "slice" apart, I have intentionally decided not to worry too much about it.

It is very painful and I can only lift my left elbow up as far as my nose, any higher and it feels like the skin would tear (which it actually did a couple of times). Whenever the scarred skin under the breast tears, it feels like a paper cut to the "tenth" degree, and then the pain can last for up to three days. I still cannot wear a bra or any fitting underwear that would touch the scar because the pain would be unbearable.

The problem of disruptive sleep has now become quite an issue. I have been trying to sleep on my back again, elevated by a few pillows so that the breast does not hang to the side. When I turn during the night, or get up to use the bathroom, it feels like a cannon ball is on my chest, moving with my body. I continue to remind myself that the worst is behind me. This encourages me to press ahead with the healing process.

I read somewhere that many cancers may be attributed to nutritional deficiencies, particularly in the area of minerals. It mentioned specifically that after surgery and treatments, we must fortify our body with the essential vitamins and minerals required to assist the healing process. I have increased my daily intake of vitamins and supplements. In addition to my daily multi-vitamin, I now take Vitamin C as well as Calcium and Vitamin D3 to help my body heal faster. I also take the Royal Bee Jelly which is a highly complex substance secreted from the glands of nursing bees. It is said to contain nutrients that are great for health and wound healing. It works for me, but everyone is different.

Doctors do not normally counsel you on nutritional and lifestyle habits post-surgery, so I made a conscious decision to do as much research as possible to help myself. One major thing I have cut out of my diet is sugar. I never consumed much sugar pre-surgery, at least, that is what I thought until I took a closer look at my sugar intake. I have had to cut out my favorite mega-sized berry juice drink on Fridays and I have drastically reduced my intake of ice cream, bakery products and chocolate bars. I now only eat the very dark chocolate, which I understand is quite beneficial to my health.

I will further reduce my intake of red meat and dairy products, although I will treat myself to a small burger and fries about once monthly, after all, I am still a "normal" human being. I am now more serious and intentional about my food choices. I do not wish to thwart or hinder my recovery.

Honey and agave are now my sweeteners of choice and I drink hot and cold, caffeine free fruit teas: ginger, lavender, chamomile, cinnamon, mint and other natural choices. I now get most of my sugar from fruits.

I will miss sugar and sugar products a lot, a whole lot. Now that I am cutting back, I am beginning to realize that I had a really well developed "sweet-tooth." Something sweet was always my special treat to myself, especially on Fridays after a hard week and although the honey is really nice, I am still going through a bit of adjustment. I have also decided to cut back substantially on wheat and corn products. This is like trying to climb Mt. Everest.

It is said that the longest journey begins with the first step—so my journey is now underway. I find that if I can hold off for about half an hour, the craving usually disappears. I ensure that fresh fruits are always in the refrigerator, so when the cravings begin, I get a slice of melon or a few berries, which help a great deal. Most times I just drink a large glass of water. The trick is to ensure there are no sweet snacks in the house. I lean on God to strengthen my will power. This is not easy.

SECTION 3

Looking Forward with Hope

ANOTHER CHRISTMAS, THANK GOD!

It is already mid-December so my surgeon advised that I let all the decisions and discussions about my "condition" wait until the New Year and he strongly urged me to throw myself into having "the best Christmas ever" and that is what I did. I began Christmas shopping, in earnest, ordering most gifts online. I thoroughly enjoy boxing, wrapping and giving gifts.

I planned my Christmas dinner and began grocery shopping. My family will arrive late Christmas Eve. I had planned the usual Christmas menu but instead of ham, I substituted two large snappers. I had to be very mindful of my dietary limitations, because during the holidays it is very tempting to cheat, so I made sure not to purchase many snack foods

I was especially looking forward to this Christmas, because in mid-August, some little shreds of doubt crossed my mind "Would I still be around?" but here I am now, filled with childish excitement.

Although my family are looking forward to the usual traditional Holiday meal that I have dutifully prepared over the years, they questioned whether I was strong enough to pull it off. My answer was a resounding "yes" as positive energy was filling my whole being. Not only was this a celebration of Christ's birth, but it was also a celebration of life for me.

We anticipated having a great time together and visiting a few friends. We will all attend my church's Christmas Day service. We are invited to a party and I have tickets for a wonderful concert. The holiday spirit has filled my home. I am looking forward to lots of laughs and making fun memories.

I began to experience some gas and bloating a few days before Christmas. I decided to go to the hospital clinic to get this situation behind me so that I could enjoy my holidays. Early on the morning of Christmas eve, I went to the clinic. While the doctor was examining me, she *slid* the stethoscope to the breast area. As it gently "hit" the scar, I felt like a thousand paper cuts had attacked my body.

When she realized my excruciating pain, she apologized profusely but it was too late. The very, very delicate skin over the scar was torn again and the damage could not be undone.

"Gas" was not my biggest issue over Christmas. The excruciating pain from the tearing of the scar was the focus of my entire physical being, but I would try my best not let it interrupt Christmas.

On returning home, I immediately took some pain killers. Being the good mother and positive person that I strive to be, I then began preparations for our casual meal tonight as well as tomorrow's Christmas dinner, with all the trimmings, but it was a Christmas of pain I would never forget.

I decided to supplement most of the appetizers and dinner sides I usually prepare, with items from my favorite deli to ease the burden of preparing so many dishes. I was proud of myself and no one noticed the difference. My "helper" (I don't like the word, "maid") worked three hours that morning, helping with the preparations and set up. I gave her a very generous bonus because without her, it would not have been possible.

Just as the radiation oncologist had warned, the itching had no respect for the festive season. On Christmas day it, along with the pain from the "thousand paper cuts" to the scar area, forced me to slow down quite a bit, but thanks to strong pain killers, my warrior spirit, and everyone pitching in, I was able to remain upbeat. I was determined not to allow this inconvenience to put a dent in my holiday festivities. Thankfully, my family never noticed my condition.

When my children were little and would fall and hurt themselves or any of the thousands of kids' mishaps, especially when having fun, I always told them, "the pain will soon go away, but you will remember the fun memories forever." I followed that advice.

Most healing is accompanied by pain. It has been four weeks now since the last radiation treatment and the pain still lingers, but I am resolute to push past the pain and submerge myself into the pleasures of this Holiday season with my family. I keep in mind that any anxiety or stress, even the good kind, may cause some interruption in healing.

I am a firm believer that our body cannot deal with increased stress and healing at the same time, so I decided, "so what if the cake stayed in the oven a tiny bit too long and got gently burnt; extra icing will take care of that, and so what if the house is a complete mess with everyone, the huge tree, the gifts, suitcases, air mattresses, etc. scattered all over, they are merely a reflection of the fun and happiness that is filling the house." So, I stepped back and allowed Christmas and New Year's Eve to happen.

I prepared a healthier meal this year. I woke up at 5:00 Christmas morning and placed the turkey in the oven to allow us to leave for church at 9:00. Upon arriving home from church, my daughter and son-in-law oven-fried two large snappers, smothered with onions, red and green bell peppers and garlic. When they removed the fish from the oven, he squeezed two large lemons over them and the fish sucked up the lemon juice and became even more succulent.

We served the fish with wild rice and veggies. I felt that the family preferred the fish to my "famous" turkey, (which they always said was the "best turkey ever") but I was very happy and not offended at all. We also prepared stuffing (especially for the kids), candied yams, but without the marshmallows, instead I rubbed a cinnamon, ginger and nutmeg mixture over them and halfway through the bake time, I drizzled a bit of maple syrup over them. We prepared a large garden salad as well. Instead of sodas, I served cold ginger tea (made with real ginger) and a strawberry lemonade (made with frozen strawberries and fresh lemons). I purchased grocery store desserts, which were a hit!

I am very grateful to God that my challenges did not spoil Christmas for the family. I was "on a mission" to ensure my grandchildren, especially, had a wonderful Christmas memory, which they all did.

Well, Christmas and New Year's Day have passed, and everyone has returned home. I survived the "dress code," but it was not easy. It was definitely an exercise in creativity and determination. The week before Christmas, after taking a very careful inventory of my light sweaters and dressy pull overs to try and find those with large collars and flaps to cover the breast area, I found myself forced to go out and purchase a few new blouses/tops to enhance my existing wardrobe, to allow me to dress appropriately for the Christmas festivities, without a bra on.

All things considered; I had an absolutely wonderful holiday filled with memories that will last forever in all our minds. I ate too much, but hey, "tis the season to be jolly" and jolly I was!

My New Year's resolution is:

God has promised that joy and happiness is always within our reach, no matter how long/short it lasts, so I have resolved to enjoy life on a daily basis. I refuse to complicate my life unnecessarily. Life is too short.
I will forgive continually and as soon as possible. I will love as God has instructed me to. I will laugh until my belly aches and I refuse to stop smiling and praising God.

It has now been five months since the surgery and six weeks since the completion of the radiation treatments. My surgeon's office called and asked me to come in. He had the results of the receptor studies which he had sent off after the surgery.

He received them some weeks prior to Christmas but with the radiation issues I was experiencing, and with Christmas upon us, he decided to wait until all the holidays were behind us, along with some of the radiation after-effects. So here I am again, waiting for the surgeon and hoping that the receptor studies went well. I am sitting sideways on the bed, table, gurney or whatever the slab of metal, rubber and cushion is called. I was looking down at my feet as they hung over the edge and, of course, there is always a long wait until the doctor "appears" so as I sat staring down at my feet, my mind began to wonder. I tried to imagine what my life would have been like these past months since the diagnosis, had the results been negative instead positive.

What would I have been doing all these lunch hours, rather than going for radiation treatments each day? Rather than having my breast fried each day, would I have been giving thanks to God for my scar free, disease free body? Would I have been thanking God for the money I would have been able to put aside, which funds I had always referred to as "not enough?"

Would I have been appreciating the ability to sleep on any side of my body that I wished? Would I have appreciated wearing a bra and any piece of clothing I wished, instead of having to sort through my closet and drawers each day for something that covers the fact that I have no bra on? Would I have been thanking him for my healthy breasts?

Would I have been thanking Him each day for guiding my life and fulfilling His promise to never leave me or forsake me and that He will care for me forever, instead of worrying incessantly about my financial future and thinking that I am in control of my life? Hmmm, I wonder. Most likely not!

I was jolted out of my thoughts when the surgeon walked in. He asked me how I was doing since our last visit and I explained about the very delicate skin over the scar area and how it was torn the day before Christmas, but he did not have any suggestions of consequence other than some insight as to why it may have happened. He prescribed a tube of antibiotic cream to put on it if it tore again and suggested that I continue to carefully monitor the area.

He then took out some notes from the file and said, "I am very pleased to advise that the receptor studies revealed that you are a candidate for hormone receptor medication." I was very happy to get that good news. In studying, I had discovered that a great number of breast cancers are estrogen-related and obviously, mine was as well.

TAMOXIFEN

He prescribed the hormone drug Tamoxifen (20 mg). Tamoxifen is the most commonly used hormone therapy for persons who have had breast cancer surgery and tested positive for estrogen receptors (ER+). Estrogen promotes the growth of breast cancer cells. Tamoxifen blocks the effects of estrogen on these cells. It is often called an "anti-estrogen" It is used to treat breast cancer. It also reduces the risk of getting cancer in the other breast. The greatest thing about the drug is that it reduces the risk of breast cancer in women who have a high risk for this disease. It is said that this drug is highly effective in lowering the risk of breast cancer recurrence. He suggested I remain on Tamoxifen for five years. We discussed possible side effects and he told me to call him if anything untoward happened.

My surgeon, like my radiation oncologist, continued to insist that my next step should be to go and consult with a medical oncologist, I cannot understand why so many specialists must deal with the same issue.

When a friend of mine had ovarian cancer, she went to a surgical oncologist, one stop shop!!!! He did everything. I sometimes wonder if all this specialty and referrals are actually money driven vs. care driven. She is now a twenty plus year survivor. Her doctor was her physician/surgeon/oncologist all wrapped up in one. When he removed her uterus, fallopian tubes and ovaries (as well as her appendix) he did what is called "an abdominal wash" (HIPEC) which is a very strong, one-time chemotherapy treatment that involves filling the abdominal cavity with chemotherapy drugs that have been heated. It is performed after the surgeon removes the organs, tumors, lesions, etc. from the abdominal area. He then prescribed estrogen inhibitor drugs for five years and that was that, twenty years ago.

The suggested medical oncologist's office is in another city which means a long day of driving to and from, beginning early in the morning and possibly not returning until late afternoon and if he needed some tests done, it may require overnighting or returning in a few days. I need some time to think about this.

FAMILY DRAMA

Speaking of stress, my son announced early on New Year's Eve that he will shortly be resigning from his job for a few months' break to "find himself and his passion so he can then enter into his true calling" My whole peace of mind went **SCREEEEECH** . . . What the heck????

I wondered how he planned to support himself and his son (he is divorced) during this sabbatical and besides in this market, jobs are very difficult to find and, in addition, he has no particular specialty. Common sense dictates that when you have a job, you stick with it unless you have a much better offer. So, what will happen when he "finds himself" but cannot find another job? He surely has no funds to start up a business.

Grown children, sometimes, cause much more stress than little ones. It was almost surreal. I heard what he said, but it was as if I was outside of my body. I took a few very deep breaths and decided that I do have choices here. Although I had no choice, at that time, in hearing what he said, because he had already spoken, I decided not to allow what he said to take over my peace of mind or ruin the holidays, I already had more than enough physical issues going on. I placed it on the back burner of my mind until the holidays were completely behind us and the New Year is firmly in place or . . . he changes his mind, whichever comes first.

For some reason, today, it popped up into my mind and I wondered what was happening with him. He had promised not "to worry me with it" so we have not spoken of it since New Year's Day and neither have the girls mentioned it since then.

I have decided against chemotherapy treatment, so I will use every bit of my energy ensuring that I am disciplined in my prayer habits, my eating habits, my exercise regimen and most importantly, I must ensure that stress does not counter-act all the good I am trying to do and that includes worrying about my grown son.

Until my surgery September past, I was a big fan of hugging. I hugged everyone I was happy to see. I loved hugs and the bigger the hug the better. I often found myself giving hugs to people I had just been introduced to, in order to break the ice. Well, during the first week in February, at a conference, I saw a wonderful friend whom I had not seen in a very long time. She is tall and beautiful, but she weighs almost 300 pounds. When we saw each other across the room, we automatically ran towards each other and as usual, embraced. OMG!! I completely forgot I cannot hug anyone yet because of my surgery. For a quick second, I forgot the flesh is still tender around the left breast area as well as the compromised bone density. Well, she grabbed me into the biggest bear hug I have ever encountered, swung me from side to side and almost squeezed the life out of me before she let me go.

Although from all outside appearances, I was totally enjoying the great, big hug, my mind immediately filled with horrible visions of bruised and/or crushed ribs from the side effects of the radiation on my rib cage, and a bruised and again swollen breast. I realized in the middle of the big hug and swing that this was a big mistake, a huge one. I immediately felt the painful pressure around the breast area and my rib cage.

That moment was the beginning of a month of concentrated pain and suffering. The pain in the entire rib cage was so intense, at times, I wondered if she had broken any bones; that was the extent of the pain. I had to constantly remind myself that the bones in that area were still very fragile from the radiation treatments and the breast was still healing.

That hug made me realize how many people hug each other during the course of a week, and especially at church. What am I going to do? I thought about it and decided that when I see a hugger coming, I will immediately position my body so that person hugs my right side. These hugs can crush "my little girl" and she screams out in pain whenever I am hugged. For the next few months, I will avoid as many parties and gatherings as possible, until the radiation after-effects and intense pain subsides.

It is now four weeks since "the hug" and the pain is only evident to the touch, not on its own strength. Praise the Lord!!! What an experience.

The Easter season is fast approaching and although I am running late this year, I am very anxious to get started on my flower gardens, outside on my front and rear balconies. I love to see the bright colors of the flowers; they brighten my days. I busied myself purchasing some Verbena, Lantana and Zinnia seedlings, as well as some Marigolds because I heard recently on TV that the Marigold plants deter mosquitos. I placed them on the front and back balconies. Thankfully, we can grow almost anything during the Spring in our climate zone, once we protect them, as much as possible, from the direct sun, keep them well watered and fertilized.

It has been a very rainy year so far, so when there is a good downpour, I collect the rainwater in various containers and then transfer it into two 5-gallon water bottles to water the plants after the rainy season has ceased. I find the rainwater nourishes the soil much better than tap water. The plants and herbs absolutely love the rainwater and flourish on it. In addition, I usually feed them every other month. I am so excited to see my garden grow and bloom right before my eyes.

I use a variety of pot sizes, shapes and colors, so the patios are very cheerful and welcoming and I get lots of compliments from the neighbors who see the cascading floral array from downstairs.

STILL PAINFUL BUT POSITIVE

I have asked God to heal my body and my mind and to forgive me of all unrighteousness and sins I have committed against Him. I know that I must listen to His word and obey it. In the Bible, our body is referred to as the temple. A temple is a holy place and should be treated accordingly, so I have made it my full-time hobby to study as much as possible about how the body works and what causes disease therein.

I have chosen not to undergo chemotherapy treatments so please note that what I am about to share is my personal opinion only and not suggested to influence anyone who might choose the medical suggestions for cancer cure/remission. We all have choices in life and this is mine.

Some years back, a friend of mine who was diagnosed with Prostate cancer decided to forgo the conventional treatments and opted for Immunotherapy treatments. After the surgery, his doctor guided him through natural lifestyle and diet changes, accompanied by the addition of extra vitamins and minerals and a water regimen that would be necessary. Six months later, my friend's PSA count went from 18 to 5 nanograms and eventually it reduced to 3.

Doctors cannot assure anyone how long they will live after cancer treatments, but up until now this sixty-eight-year-old professional tennis player feels absolutely great and is healthy. When I spoke with him recently, he promised to send me a copy of the guideline booklet he received from his doctor and, upon receipt, I read it right away. The information was excellent and I immediately began to follow the lifestyle and diet guidelines noted therein, along with information I gathered from a few other sources.

My extensive research highlighted some possible situations that may cause cancer to invade our bodies and also explained the great importance of balance in our lives. Balance is something that most of us lack in this rat race of a stressed-out life so many of us live. As I had already read in the Bible, my research reiterated that until we are able to free our minds of all hate, envy, anger, regret, bitterness, anxiety, jealousy, doubt and fear, there is nothing that any diet or exercise regimen can do to assist heal our body. I found out that stress causes our blood to become acidic and cancer thrives in an acidic environment.

Our first order of business should be to work diligently on our mind and emotions. We have to dig deep, really, really deep and ascertain the root cause of the anxiety. In many instances, stress causes our muscles to become tense and stiff and also affects our bowel functions. So many of us allow family drama, finances, our jobs, our anger with ex-persons in our life, jealousy, etc. to rob us of a full night's sleep. Even though we may easily fall off to sleep, we sometimes find ourselves waking up after a few hours and cannot relax our racing minds enough to allow us to fall back into any manner of "sweet" slumber.

We must convince ourselves that we can get out of this rut we have gotten ourselves into. We must truly believe that with God on our side, all things are possible, in accordance with His perfect will for our lives. We must rebuke the spirit of defeat. That is our only option when we are down in the trenches of life. We either raise up or sink further down. All day long we must ask God to hold on tightly to us, because if we hold on to Him our grip may slip, but with Him holding on to us, we are always protected.

We must go on a mission to free our minds and soul of all the negativity that we have carried around for so many years. In so many instances, we also pass along stress to our children. Many babies are being born unwell due to the mother's stress level and other negative lifestyles during pregnancy.

Life lesson: I will keep in mind that although things around me sometimes seem to be imploding, I will stand firm and claim the victory that God has promised me. I will allow His presence and promises to be my comfort and my strength. I will closely follow the guidance in His word for my life.

When we eventually decide to forgive others, and most especially our own selves, we realize that we have no power over what others have already done to us and how others feel about us. When we put the bitterness and fear and anger behind us, then and only then can we begin the work of converting our chronically sick and acidic blood to an alkaline and healthy environment that is conducive to healing our diseases.

Since, apparently it is difficult for cancer to thrive in an alkaline environment, I set out to learn how I can change my blood PH to a more alkaline state, while de-cluttering my mind. Human blood PH should be very slightly alkaline (everything in balance) An acidic PH can occur from eating acid forming foods as well as emotional stress. This deprives the cells of the vital oxygen that they require. An acidic PH also decreases the body's ability to absorb minerals and other nutrients and decreases energy production in the cells.

I read that our diets should consist of approximately 60% alkaline forming foods and only 40% of acid forming foods. Until our health is restored, we may need to take additional vitamins and trace minerals which help build up our immune system. One of the vitamins suggested was Vitamin D3 (in capsule form) which apparently is a great immune system booster as well as a big help in improving bone health. Sunshine is also a great supplier of natural Vitamin D and it is pure and free.

An older (and very healthy) friend of mine suggested that an excellent way to help clear out some of the acidity from my body is to squeeze half a lemon/or a whole one (if you wish) into a glass of warm water each morning and drink it fifteen minutes before I eat or drink anything else. I have heard this many times over the years, but paid no real attention to it. You can also do this prior to your evening meal if you so desire. Each morning I drink a warm glass of water with a squeezed lemon in it. It is now a part of my morning routine.

About fifteen minutes later I eat two servings of fruit and then two slices of gluten free bread, toasted, with my home-made blueberry jam, made with honey instead of sugar. Sometimes I also smear a few drops of pure virgin olive oil on the toast as well. This is a way to get your natural oils which the body needs instead of the hydrogenated oils.

You may be asking, but aren't lemons and limes acidic?—yes, they are, but when they enter our digestive system, the natural juices in our stomach render them alkaline, so no worry there. I have increased my water intake to the suggested eight glasses per day and that has surely helped with the elimination of toxins and other waste from my body.

I am ashamed to say I never really knew my blood type, never had any reason to, I guess, but then a friend bought me a book for Christmas regarding ***Your Blood Type and your Diet***. I read it and found it to be interesting, so I went and had my blood tested and discovered I am B Positive. I then re-read the sections of the book that referred to my blood type and realized, for the most part, I was already eating in accordance with my blood type, so I felt good about that.

I accept that my healing is totally in God's hands and according to His will for me. I am going to do everything humanly possible to ensure I am doing my share of what is right for my body, mind and soul as laid out in His word.

Note to self: I have heard many times over the years: "Do your best and God will do the rest" So that is what I am striving to do.

I recently treated myself to a juicing machine. I make pure juice from my favorite fruits and vegetables, i.e. carrots, apples, kiwi, cucumbers, celery, kale and parsley at least twice per week. A friend of mine does this every day, but my machine is difficult to clean, so I can only manage to do it on the weekends. I really enjoy the juice, especially realizing that it is instantly absorbed into the blood cells and begins cleansing and healing within half an hour. When I drink a glass of "juice" I realize I am getting a mega dose of natural vitamins and essential minerals directly into my blood stream—with no sweeteners, additives or preservatives. I eat lots of green leafy vegetables as well because they are incredibly good for the immune system and the blood.

Since I have made these small, simple changes, I have already started to feel much healthier and my quality of life has improved, and especially, I now sleep without pills. I still desire deeper sleep, but I am much better than I was before. I have decided that no matter my life span, I will continue to do my best to keep my temple in the best condition I possibly can as it has real time benefits.

CHEMOTHERAPY OR NOT

It is now mid-March and I am checking in at the reception desk of the medical oncologist of my choice. Why did I wait three months? Well, after carefully considering the pros and cons of the one I was recommended to see, I did some research and chose a local, but well-respected one instead.

As I sit waiting in his inner office, many scary thoughts filled my mind, but I prayed them away. My thoughts were interrupted when the door opened and a handsome, athletic looking young doctor walked in. He had a pleasant demeanor.

The questions begin and I tell him, up front, I do not wish to undergo any chemotherapy treatments. For a few seconds, his face registered shock, especially as chemotherapy is his specialty. I could read his face and it was asking, "why then are you here?" I told him that I had promised my surgeon and my radiation oncologist that I would "have a talk" with him. He was familiar with both my doctors. I did not mention, however, that they both recommended another medical oncologist. I handed him copies of my file. He continued to ask questions about my medical history, my lifestyle, etc. and I continued to give him all the information I could recall. He then took a few minutes to review the file I had brought from my surgeon.

After a while he asked me to excuse him and he went into another office for about fifteen minutes. I spent the time he was away thinking about all the patients that he had attended to but had lost to death and I wonder how that affects his psyche. I guess his balance and satisfaction are found in those patients who survive.

When he returned, he had about four pages of graphs in his hands. He placed them, all highlighted in red and green, in front of me. He had taken all of the information that he had obtained from me and from my file and placed it into the computer, which had sorted it into segments and then spewed out the graphs. These graphs showed what the computer app felt were my chances of survival if I did/did not do certain things, and based on my past health history, it noted what it felt I could expect and the time frames thereof, going forward. I smiled as I glanced at them, because, after all, what does a computer know about the real issues in my life and even more so, what God has in store for me.

I was rather uncomfortable with all their impersonal graphs and possibly, erroneous results. One of these days, an oncologist who has personally survived cancer should write a book for his colleagues about how to interact with cancer patients and what type of bedside manner to use when dealing with already sick, scared patients.

Mind you, this doctor was very attentive, he took his time, he was patient with me in getting the information he required but he was a bit taken aback when all the computer information he provided did not seem to intimidate me.

History suggests that the world and everything in it is rapidly evolving and when we look back over the past fifty to one hundred years at some of the treatments and remedies that were popular back then, but are now banned or no longer in use today (for obvious reasons) I shudder to think about the thousands of persons who may have died because of those same, at the time, popular medicines/treatments.

Technology, information sharing, research and science have evolved dramatically since then and will continue to evolve and I am personally convinced that chemotherapy, in its present form, will eventually be discontinued and some other less invasive and less poisonous form of cancer cure will replace it.

I sincerely believe that even in my lifetime, this breakthrough will be introduced and I will look back and rejoice that God blessed me and guided me away from it at this time. At the end of the visit, he suggested that I go home and read up on all the information he gave me and think carefully about my options (as per the computer graph) and return in three weeks.

In the meantime, I had begun to experience neck problems again. My neck would hurt each morning I awoke and even some times during the day. After a while it became quite painful. Again, I went to the clinic and had an X-ray done, only to discover that the neck vertebrae had deteriorated quite a bit since my last visit. The missing cartilage obvious around the area was unbelievable. She did not give me any medicine for it but suggested that I buy a new mattress and most definitely a new and more functional pillow. I surely had no funds for a new mattress so I went out and tested about 10 pillows before I settled on one that cost $150. Hmmm, one night down and I cannot feel any improvement, but I guess it takes time.

A few weeks later, I started to feel a painful lump in my throat. As you can imagine, after being twice misdiagnosed, I take no chances. I dashed off to the ENT doctor who said it had something to do with my neck's existing problem of osteopenia and he ordered quite a number of allergy tests (whatever for I do not understand) but in any event, the allergy results came back a few days later stating, basically, the same thing the blood type book had stated, and top of the list was that I should not be eating any corn or corn products at all. Are they serious? I have been trying, but do they realize that corn is in everything? What am I to eat, I wonder?

Apparently, I am also allergic to peanuts and while I love them, I can live without them, but all corn products? It also mentioned oranges and one or two other fruits, but I will pay no attention to that part of it for now, I love oranges too much. It seems another battle begins . . . the nutritional battle against what I love to eat, what my body is allergic to and what it needs to thrive on.

Is it just me, or does everyone reading this book visit some type of doctor almost every month? What next, I wonder?

Goal: Today I pledge to use my faith like an arrow and shoot it towards my target of healing and a wonderful future filled with blessings and fulfillment of God's promises.

It has now been five months since my son "retired" and in those months, he has considered everything from opening a barbeque Joint, a game room, to an automotive parts retail shop. Last month, he asked if he could "borrow" some money from me to pay his son's monthly child support. I decided I did not want my grandson to suffer, so I personally sent the money to the ex-wife.

Yesterday, he was threatened with eviction and his landlord, who is a close family friend, called my younger daughter asking that she encourage him to pay up or he has no choice but evict him and place his belongings in storage.

My daughter called me screaming. She said that it was very embarrassing to have the landlord call her and then to make matters worse, when she called my son to find out his side of the story, he was blaming the landlord because, he said the landlord had no right to expose his personal matters to anyone. While that may be true, the landlord, I am sure, was only trying to help him. My daughter and son got into a big "fight" and she hung up on him.

The initial announcement of the sabbatical caused my mind to go **SCREEECH!!** Now, I can no longer keep it on the back burner. I called my son and he rambled on about how one cannot get evicted without proper prior notice and that his landlord has not given him the requisite official notice and required time frame. "Are you serious?" I asked, "are you blaming the landlord because your sabbatical plans have gone down the toilet? What does your personal financial problems have to do with the landlord?"

He continued to ramble on. "I will bunk with a friend for a while until I can get settled." "The challenge," he continued, "is to find somewhere to store my belongings in the meantime." My son was definitely not referring to a storage facility; he was referring to some family or friend's garage or shed. I became terribly upset. I could not believe that all these years of hard work and dedication to his career had ended up like this. If you remember, he did not discuss this decision to resign, with the family. He made this decision without consulting anyone. Now he is trying to get help from anyone who is willing to give him a hand-out.

For a few days, I fumed inwardly and then I realized that my son and his problems were coming in between me and my worship and peace of mind, so I had to "shake it loose." I refuse to allow him to come in between me and my faith in God. It was not easy. Not easy at all. He is, of course, my son and I love him very much, but obviously he cares only about himself and his personal desires. If he cared about his own son, he would have rethought his decision and surely if he had spent any time, at all, in thought about how this could negatively impact my peace of mind, he may have considered other options. In the end, it was all about HIM, and no one else.

I went into my own "faith boot camp" and after about a week, I was able to shake off worrying about my son and his life. I am in my own battle and I cannot fight two battles at the same time. I chose to defer to God and His will for him. I constantly pray that God will deliver him from whatever hole he has dug for himself, but I cannot allow any of my physical or emotional or faith energy to be wasted on a 33-year-old man who single handedly, made a conscious choice to mess up his life.

Lesson to self: If you truly believe in God and His perfect will for
your life, you would believe that He will take on all your cares
and concerns and work them all for the best, in His time.

I love my job and I have the best "boss" ever. I know and adore her family, as well. She has been there with me through this entire journey and has been very liberal in allowing me to attend doctor visits. She ensures that I am not over worked. She has been my rock!

Working in a small office can be a good thing but it can also be not so good at times. We all sit in one large space with a few executive offices along the outer wall (with windows) and the remainder of us sit in cubicles or in open spaces. In this setting there is absolutely no privacy and if someone is having a bad day (or bad night before and brought it to work) then we are all exposed to that person's "wrath."

One particular executive envies my relationship with my boss and the staff, in general. She is in a bad marriage, feels insecure among her siblings (all of whom are successful, with relatively good marriages, and are comfortable in their own skins) so she desperately seeks affirmation from the employees, via power of her office, to validate her self-worth. With her, you never know what to expect, she swings from hysterically happy to extremely angry in any given hour. Today, I was her victim. I was the object of her hunger for power and recognition.

My supervisor was at a day-long Conference so the senior executive asked me to send out an e-mail on behalf of my supervisor. The e-mail was to go to our Head office advising them of a proposal that our department wished to initiate. As is the accepted protocol, I copied my supervisor and the senior executive who gave me the instructions. A vicious member of the department told the "troubled" executive that I had directly communicated with head office. Well, she ran into the senior executive's office and began to rant and rave.

"How could Mrs. Isador, a mid-level member of the staff, send out an e-mail directly to head office, without consulting me or including me in the list of recipients," she complained.

"You are not a part of that particular project or in any way involved with that department. There's no reason for you to have been included," responded the senior executive.

"I do not think a 'junior' staff member should not be sending out e-mails to the head office without including me, a senior member of staff." Blah, Blah, Blah . . .

Of course, this "problem" swept through our little office like wildfire and I became the brunt of the latest office gossip.

When the senior executive later spoke to me about it, I said "That's water off my back. I only did as I was told to do by you, so if she has a problem, it's not with me." Later on, that evening, however, my thoughts reverted to the incident and I replayed it in my mind and I became quite upset and it took all of my calming skills to settle down to sleep.

My direct supervisor is back today, and I am sure she will hear about it, but it will not be from me as I will not regurgitate this petty bit of office politics. If she asks me about it, I will refer her to the senior executive who approached me to dispatch the e-mail and let them deal with it. My time is far too precious to get involved in office poli-tricks.

ONE YEAR POST SURGERY

It has now been one year since the official medical diagnosis, however, in real time it is actually one month short of two years since my personal diagnosis and trips to the doctor and the imaging lab for confirmation and being told that "nothing is the matter."

The good news is that it is one year since the surgery and eight months since completion of the radiation. My thoughts? I am very grateful and thankful to be alive and still functioning fully at work and being able to praise the Lord for His healing, His mercies and forgiveness. I still have pains in the breast area (apparently this is the norm with a lumpectomy as well as post radiation treatments). I am still unable to wear a bra full time, because of the very fragile and delicate skin covering the scar which runs from the nipple down to at least two inches along the wall of the chest. I have to live with the scarring and the unnatural fragility of the scar caused by the radiation. Any pressure on the area causes the skin to tear very easily.

Whenever I absolutely have to wear a bra, although I ensure it is loose fitting; after a while, it feels as if the skin over the scar area has been burned by fire. The skin under the area is as fragile now as it was in December past when it was accidently torn by the doctor's stethoscope. In an attempt to ease this problem, I purchased some large non-abrasive band-aids to cover/protect the scar area when I have to wear a bra. The band-aids help for up to about two hours, after which time the pressure of the bra's band under the breast, still causes discomfort.

Sometimes the other breast hurts as well, and once in a while I still get shooting pains in my upper arm, between my elbow and the shoulder blade, as well as in my armpit, just under the area from where the lymph nodes were removed.

During a recent visit to my surgeon I mentioned that sometimes I have bouts of shortness of breath and even dizziness especially when exercising and he advised that they could possibly be side effects of the Tamoxifen drug I am taking. I went home and read up on the possible side effects and for the most part, I feel lucky that I did not experience any other of the side effects noted, except for hair thinning, so I no longer concerned myself with it, but it is good to know the feelings were nothing unrelated to the medicine.

For my summer vacation this year, me and my grandchildren are spending a week up north at a lake front resort community. Our family has vacationed there a few times over the years. The weather was wonderful the afternoon we arrived. Later that evening we went to a "Grill and Chill" party sponsored by the resort and by the time we arrived back at the cabin around 10:00 pm, we were so exhausted from flying and unpacking and the party, we could barely stay awake.

We planned an action-packed week. We swam, "tried" to paddle-board, hiked, fished, in fact, we did everything we love to do. Some days we packed lunches and snacks and spent the entire day outdoors having all the fun we could possibly muster up. Some evenings, if we wished to eat at home, we would make wonderful and fun dinners, especially on the outside grill, then we would play board games, word games and just enjoy chatting about the frolics of the day. It was a wonderful time of bonding and we took some great pictures to serve as reminders of how much we love each other's company and the wonderful hills and the lake community we enjoy so dearly. I usually compile three photo albums for the grandkids to share with their parents.

The following week after returning home, I began to experience some really intense pain in my chest area, my ribs and the muscles of my lower abdomen just above my left thigh. It was so intense that I began to harbor thoughts of cancer invading other areas of my body, but I was determined not to go running to the doctor again. I took pain killers in the mornings so I could perform efficiently at work during the day and again at night so I could get to sleep. I prayed constantly and eventually quieted my crazy thoughts.

I decided the pains were from the extreme amount of physical activity: climbing, swimming, walking and everything hikers, campers and swimmers do. After a while I decided to use cold/warm compresses and hot showers to get some relief, instead of taking the pain medication at night.

Another area of my life that has changed relates to the amount of pain medication I took pre-diagnosis. Since becoming an adult, my sinuses have become increasingly annoying and I have been on some type of sinus and/or pain medication, off and on, for the majority of my adult life. Since this health challenge and especially because I take the drug Tamoxifen daily, I have decided to decrease the amount of pain (or sinus) medication unless it is a real emergency, and this is an emergency, for now, that is.

Three weeks later the pain still persisted. I finally gave in and went to see my new primary care doctor who sent me for an MRI. A week later I returned to his office and he showed me the results and explained that everything was in order. As I had suspected, the pains were a result of the strenuous activity on my vacation. He said that any overactivity could cause pain in the upper portion of my body due to the after-effects of the radiation, and he advised me to keep that in mind because it was possible the radiation could have caused some compromise of the bone density in that area. He suggested I continue to do regular exercises, rotate the cold and hot compresses and in case of severe pain, to take some aspirin and eventually the pains should cease. He reminded me that I was still sick and not yet "out of the woods"

When I decided to take this vacation with the grandkids, there were three things I obviously did not take into consideration, firstly I am no longer in the first half of my life, and secondly, anything done to any extreme, can cause dire consequences. Additionally, I did not take into account that my body had undergone surgery and radiation and some weakening over the last year.

"Will I ever be the strong person I was, pre surgery?" I asked myself. I decided to make a change. I will gradually increase my daily exercise regimen, slowly and gently, but regularly. As well, I will never spend an entire week of constant swimming, climbing and walking up hills ever again. I will pace myself more sensibly next time.

I waited another six weeks before I returned to the medical oncologist's office. I told him that I was experiencing pains in my lower left abdomen. He pressed and prodded and pressed again and said that he cannot feel anything that I should be concerned about. After further examination of the other areas of concern, and much more discussion about my refusal to undergo chemotherapy, he ordered a slew of blood work including a CEA, CA 125 and CA 27.29 as well as an Oncotype DX which, among other things, I understand, is supposed to show whether I need chemotherapy treatments or not. He also wrote up a prescription for a mammogram and an Ultrasound.

The Onco test cost about $5,000 with a $1,000 co-pay, in addition to the regular copay for the visit. I was most surprised to discover that I was charged an extra cost for the nurse to extract the blood from my veins. This disease is very costly. I cannot help but wonder what happens to those persons who do not have Insurance and also those who cannot afford the co-pays.

I cannot believe we have come to the point where there is an additional charge for the nurse to draw the blood from my veins? In my past experiences, that procedure was always included in the cost of the visit, but obviously this medical oncologist did not subscribe to those rules.

Again, I wonder what I would I have done with all this money that I have personally spent on this disease this past year, had I not been diagnosed. It is difficult to believe that at the beginning of this journey, I labeled myself as "broke" and was very apprehensive regarding my future financial outlook. At this moment in time, my future financial outlook is absolutely the last thing on my mind. My new goal is now to arrive at the future instead of worrying about the financial aspect thereof.

As I very casually add up what I have personally spent on treatments/visits/medicines not covered by the Insurance, on deductibles, co-pays, etc. over the past year, I realize that there is no way I would have saved that amount. This tells me that we all can do a much better job at putting aside funds than we presently do. Isn't it amazing how we are able to come up with the deductibles, co-pays and all the other related expenses but could not, otherwise, in the normal course, have saved that same amount of money?

Life lesson: We can always save more than we think we can.

My whole outlook on life has changed. Sometimes I step back from the crowd and observe people as they speak of what they will be doing next year, the next five and ten years. They exude such confidence and assurance. I just smile, because they have no idea what tomorrow could bring. I recall doing the same thing just two years ago, before the course of my life was changed by the cancer diagnosis.

Everything I wish to have or to do, is now predicated on the realization that only God knows if I will live to see tonight, next week or next year. While I continue to have high hopes and wonderful dreams for my future, now I hold on to them more loosely. One pain or discomfort could turn my life completely around and dispel every hope and dream I have.

Many of my friends and colleagues, in various stages of the disease, tried every possible treatment, every herbal remedy, but still died from cancer. I am now convinced that we will never understand why some persons succumb so easily, whereas others, even some who are gravely ill, survive. No doctor, medicine, diet plan, exercise regimen, nothing can ensure survival. Only God knows the plans He has for each of us; and only each patient, personally, knows how much they really want to survive to the other side of this cancer. Accepting the fact that I could possibly be on borrowed time, I will do everything in my power to ensure my health is at its best. But along the way,

I will occasionally indulge in a slice of chocolate cake, although it is said that white flour is bad for me.

I will order that medium-well Porterhouse steak, with lots of onions, when the occasion presents itself, or just because I want to.

I will have a scoop of strawberry or coffee ice-cream once in a while, to please my taste buds.

Yes, I will have that occasional Margarita or glass of wine to celebrate a happy occasion.

Yes, I will wear every item of clothes in my closet instead of waiting for that illusive "special occasion."

And Yes, I continue to invest in making wonderful memories with those I love.

Next year I hope to take my grandchildren on a rail tour halfway across the country, stopping along the way and enjoying everything each state has to offer, especially in the culinary area and taking in all the history and facts we can along the way. Yes, I am making plans for the future, cautiously, of course.

This is my hope and my dream for 2014. If it is God's will, it will happen, if not, then either I will be on the way to, or already arrived into the arms of Jesus. One way or the other, what will be will be. But in the meantime, I will make sure that every minute of this gift of life I have now, is enjoyed to the fullest.

I refuse to be unhappy,
I refuse to sit back and cry,
I refuse to be sad,
I refuse to be lonely,
I refuse to look back,
I refuse to apologize for my extravagant enjoyment of each day of my life,
I refuse to put anything off for later that I can do in the present.

I have determined that only lack of opportunity, time or money will deter me from maximizing this chance at life that God has now blessed me with. No doubts or fears about my health, finances or my future will slow me down or make me waste valuable time worrying.

I refuse to worry about what others think about me.
I refuse to allow the negative words of others, to get inside of me.
I refuse to miss one family gathering or the celebration of a birthday of a dear friend.
I refuse to be a spectator in life. I want to be fully involved whenever I am afforded the opportunity.
I refuse to overthink the possibility of death, because accidents/heart attacks/ strokes/diseases can happen to even the most unlikely persons. Every one of us is already in the line-up, unaware of when it will be our time.
I refuse to rethink or over analyze any of God's promises to me.
I receive them all and I hold on to all of them, no matter what His will is for me.

I will go out every morning looking forward to the best that the day has to offer me, expecting good health and His blessings to fill me to overflowing.

Journal entry: Until the day of my exit from this earth, I expect the absolute best that God has in store for me.

I want the lessons I have learned along this cancer journey to enable me to help others in their walk.

I believe that God forgives all my sins and that His Holy Spirit surrounds me, leads me and guides me to His face eventually.
I expect healing, physical and spiritual, because I believe . . .
I believe that only good will come from this experience and however long or short term it lasts, my testimony will give life and encouragement to others.
I believe.

I am comforted in the fact that I have been blessed with fifty-eight wonderful years so far and that I have a loving family, a great church family, many dear friends and an abundance of wonderful memories.

I fully expect to live long enough to make many more.
I am determined that each day, I will make someone's day "their best day."
I thank God daily for what He has already done in my life and I thank Him, in advance, for what He will do for me and those I love.
I will thank Him when I am in pain and I will thank Him when I am doing perfectly well. I will praise His Holy name the entire day long, when I arise in the morning, when I am driving to work and I will praise him at work.
I will constantly brag about His blessings in my life. I do not always understand His ways or His timing or His will, but I will trust that He loves me and will protect me from all harm and danger.

I have come to know and appreciate that just as He is with me in my mountain top experiences, He is just as present in the valley experiences of my life.

He has promised that when we go through the valley, He will be with us. Note, He said going through, not stopping in the valley. In my valley experiences, I will hold on even tighter, so He can guide me towards His light. I look to Him, only, for my help and guidance. "With God, all things are possible, if we believe."

Most people, when they are overcome by life's problems and fears, they head to the phone and call friends and family, hoping that someone can advise/ encourage them and eventually solve their problems. When medical problems arise, they rush to the phone to call their medical professionals. All this is good, we all need the support of family and friends and medical professionals but, my advice is, in future, before you rush to the phone, rush to the Throne. The Throne of God should be your first stop. God will guide us to the next stop.

I will ensure I am being the best I can be and remain alert and as careful as I can. That is common sense. In reality I do not have enough funds for the retirement I always dreamed of, especially now. But I know that He is with me. He has promised to always take care of my needs, so I do not worry about that aspect of my future anymore. I will do my part and spend wisely.

There are lots of things about life that I still do not understand and even some that appear, on the surface, to be unfair. I will not concern myself with it. I will, however, trust Him to always be there for me, no matter what.

I will not wait until I am cancer free for five years to share my experience because I believe that I have a real message of encouragement and faith to share now with those going through similar circumstances. I journal everything and will share this experience with anyone willing to listen. I thank God for the many lives I will touch, encourage and be an example to, I will remind them of how important reliance on God really is.

Each morning I awake, there is a song in my heart. I am always amazed at which song pops up. I then sing more praises to Him, no matter if I am in pain or not—that does not matter, because despite the pain, I am perfectly at peace and whole in my spirit. God has not given up on me and I will not stop praising Him. He is an awesome God and worthy of my constant praise. He loves me unconditionally.

This is now my third visit to the medical oncologist's office. It took just over a month before all the results were in his office and I was called in to discuss them with him. Apparently, the lab sent some results that were not requested and did not perform some of the tests that were requested; they had to be redone. So here I am sitting in the waiting room and as you can imagine, this is when your faith is truly tested. What will the results reveal? What hand has God dealt me with regards these past two years of suffering and hoping. I tried to stay calm, but my human self was all in a tizzy.

I had the first appointment and when I arrived, I was the only person in the waiting room, so I tried watching TV, but that did not work. I had to wait at least 30 minutes before the doctor was able to see me. In the meantime, it seems as if I read every magazine, every newspaper, every pamphlet and of course, I could not recall any of what I was reading. Just drawing blanks.

One by one, bald headed women and sick looking men came into the Waiting room. In the normal course, this environment does nothing for your self-esteem, but when I noticed how sick some of the patients appeared, I am thankful that I was spared what they seem to be suffering. Again, I rely on the Word, "In all things, with prayer and supplication, giving thanks"

Just then, my name was called and I hurried into the doctor's office. I do not know if my haste was to quickly separate myself from the persons in the waiting room or to rush to get the results, which my faith was telling me to be confident about. Here it is, my faith speaking in one ear and my human nature shouting in the other ear. What a battle.

I was feeling very healthy. I was not allowing the occasional pain to be a cause of worry, so I had high hopes that everything was going to be great. We exchanged the usual pleasantries and he began to read, to himself, the results received from the lab. He then realized that the Oncotype DX test results, which had to be re-ordered, were still not into his office, after all this time. Excusing himself, he said "I am going to have my technician call the lab and ask them to immediately fax over the results, if, in fact, they have completed them." So again, I am by myself.

I saw him go into another office to see a patient, in the meantime. If nothing else, this whole experience has taught me to be patient. He eventually returned with the faxed results and he began to quietly read and re-read all of them.

Before he discussed the results, he asked "How are you feeling, today?" "Excellent, except for the occasional pain and discomfort in my breast area." I did mention that the pain in my lower left abdomen was still a bit of an issue, although not constant, it has not yet disappeared completely. He suggested that I go and see my surgeon for a further opinion. He then read the results of the cancer/tumor marker blood tests received and confirmed that all the results were good.

When he arrived at the results of the Oncotype DX, he pushed the forms over so that I could read them with him. He said, "See this figure here, this indicates where you stand. 10 is where you are on this scale. This is because you are what is referred to as 'Node Positive' meaning that the cancer had already leaked into the lymph nodes." I did not understand the parameters of the scale, so in my world, 10 was the maximum. A quickly sinking feeling encompassed my being but I was able to maintain an outward appearance of calm.

He then went on to explain that it was 10 out of 50. "Whew, thank God," I thought. He pointed to the line on the graph which indicated the mortality rate if I chose not to take the chemotherapy treatments as well as the line on the graph indicating the mortality rate if I *did choose* to take chemotherapy treatments.

He looked at me for a moment to see if I was grasping the information. Was he kidding? I had no idea whatsoever what he was showing me, other than 10 out of 50 was not a bad result. The graph lines meant nothing to me. I could not (or would not) assimilate any of the information outlined.

After more discussion, he said, "Mrs. Isador, based on the results, there would be NO substantial benefit to you undergoing chemotherapy treatments."

He continued, "While the graph shows a slight benefit to taking the treatment, it is minimal, and not worth it at this time."

I asked myself, "Is he saying that my choice not to poison myself was the right choice? Had I not taken the Onco test, would I ever have known that?" I wondered if all cancer patients are required to take the Onco test prior to receiving chemo treatments.

If I had listened to the urging of my doctors and just blindly gone ahead with the treatments, I might have completed, at least, the first round by now. BUT GOD . . . spoke and I listened.

I listened to the urging of God, that He is able to use my body to heal itself, with or without the chemotherapy as He saw fit.

"Oh my God, how can I express my Thanks for what you have done?" I feel very vindicated. I followed the Holy Spirit's lead which was the best decision for my life.

I jumped up from my chair and hugged the doctor. I wanted to do flips in the office and scream "THANKS BE TO GOD" the creator and architect of my life.

Please note, I am not suggesting anything here; again, I am just sharing my personal experience. Everyone and each case are different. This is how I, personally, was led by the Holy Spirit.

He smiled. "Congratulations! I suggest regular follow up visits of every three months for the time being, to ensure everything remains on track," he said. "Everything relating to the breast cancer is going just fine."

I could not contain myself. My body felt as if it was exploding with happiness and validation. Words cannot express my joy.

I paid the bill, arranged the follow up visit and floated to my car. In the car, I turned up the volume of my praise music and drove from the parking lot on to the main road. I shouted praises all the way back to my office. I was very excited!

I could not wait for later; immediately as I returned to my desk, I sent e-mails to my family and the friends with whom I had shared this journey. I promised to call them after work.

When I finished work that evening, the excitement had not diminished. I jumped into my car, drove along the waterfront and sang until I did not recognize any of the buildings or streets around me. I then turned around and drove the eight miles back home. My faith was validated. Only God . . .

I was overcome with joy. I wanted to jump up and down and shout praises to the heavens all night. It took a few days for me to fully digest what had just happened. I had followed my heart and the urging of The Holy Spirit, refused chemotherapy, survived without it and received confirmation that I had made the right choice.

I called both my doctors and shared the good news with them. They were happy for me.

My next step was to make an appointment with my surgeon to determine what is causing this discomfort in my lower left abdomen. The medical oncologist did not deal with it to any extent. I am not overly concerned because all the blood work, scans and tumor markers remain encouraging! I just want to understand why the pain is still lingering.

The enormity of my blessings hit me later that evening when I got word that a dear friend of mine who had late stage bone cancer, was losing the battle. I was lost for words. He was one of the most athletic men I ever met, with a first-class attitude toward life.

A few years back, he had tried to jump over a barrier wall, but did not quite make it and his lower back landed on the top edge of the wall. Although he realized that he had injured himself, and was in a lot of pain, he decided that the situation did not warrant medical attention, so he never checked with a doctor to ascertain the extent of the damage.

A year after the fall, the pain became so debilitating he was forced to seek medical attention. He was unable to walk completely upright. The doctor discovered he had crushed three of his vertebrae during the accident. He ordered a bone scan of the entire spinal column, in addition to other blood tests to determine his general physical condition. The tests revealed that he had developed early stage bone cancer. He underwent surgery for the crushed vertebrae. After a lengthy recovery period, he continued his exercise regimen, became a vegetarian and went on with his life.

I found out later that he did not return to the doctor after the surgery and took no medication for the cancer for the next two years. Unbelievable!

Early last year, however, the pain became so unbearable, he was forced to consult with his doctor. His test results revealed that the cancer had progressed to Stage 4.

It is now four years since the accident and one year since he has begun cancer treatment. During this past year, he has been experiencing the most excruciating pain, suffering and undergoing radical medical procedures. He has endured several rounds of chemotherapy and radiation. He receives regular blood transfusions to keep his cell count up. The whole ordeal and the intense pain have left him quite weak. His movements have become progressively slower. Some days the pain is so intense, he can barely speak. Realizing that this situation is his own fault, he blames no one but is now holding on to God's promise never to leave him or forsake him. He has attributed his survival, so far, to God's mercy. Everyone is different and entitled to make their own life choices. I have not reprimanded him in any way.

He had told me that, until recently, he walked each morning, did push-ups and weight training, all in a herculean effort to build up his bone strength. His attitude is unbelievable, he is a natural comedian. He finds humor in everything around him. He especially laughs at himself. He tells of how, whenever he goes to the oncology clinic, the nurses and other healthcare professionals all begin to smile, just in anticipation of the jokes he will share while he is being attended to, or the stories he will tell about what is happening/or not, in his life nowadays.

He said his doctors are amazed by him. They only expected him to live for six months after the stage 4 bone cancer diagnosis. At times, he makes suggestions to the doctors for some new or alternative treatment. They are always baffled at his knowledge and his winning spirit. They are amazed that he is still mobile and in such high spirits, considering his pain and suffering. They refer to him as "The Miracle Man." He looks forward to his visits to the clinic where he always encourages the other patients.

Last week, he and his wife, who now does all the driving, visited me. When I remarked how well he looked and how strong he seemed to be, physically and emotionally, he assured me that as long as there is life in his body, he will praise the Lord. Whether he has to encourage others from a wheelchair, on crutches, in a waiting room or from a hospital bed, he will enjoy every minute of his life and be a light to all those around him.

While death is inevitable, he pledged to do whatever he can, for as long as he can to enjoy his time with family and friends. He refuses to lie about and wait for this disease to overtake him and knock him down. His situation has really made me realize that only God knows and controls our time on this earth. Only He determines the date of our entrance, how this life will play out for us, and the date of our exit.

THE CLOUDS

As I lay in my bed that September night, thinking and praying I saw, out of the corner of my eye, a very bright light streaming in from outside the window. I got up, went over to the window, and before I could open the blinds further, my eyes feasted on the most beautiful and the brightest full moon I have ever seen. I stood transfixed for quite a while, just enjoying God's magnificent creation. It had completely lit up the sky. After quite a while, with the blinds still open, I went back into bed where I still had a great view of that majestic scene.

Then, in the blink of an eye, utter blackness replaced the silver glow of the moon. For a while, I questioned my sanity, then I jumped out of bed and again went over to the plate glass window, through which I could have a much clearer view of the sky. Then it hit me, large, billowing black clouds had quickly and totally obscured my view of the beautiful, bright moon. The clouds had come between me and the moon.

As I continued to stand there watching the now black sky, I noticed that, ever so slowly, light began to show up from behind the dark clouds and within minutes the brilliant and beautiful moon was once again in full view. This fascinated me! I continued to stand there and watch the moon show up and disappear, time after time, quite like a game of hide and seek.

Suddenly, it occurred to me that this was a wonderful revelation from God. This was a reminder of His promise that He would never leave us or forsake us. The clouds of life will come and seem to overtake His glory, protection and promises, BUT behind every dark cloud that comes into our life, God is still right there, in full brilliance and with full power. His mercy is endless, His grace never diminishes, His word never fades away, no matter what cloud comes between us and Him.

From now on, during the hard times, the times when I find myself in a dark place and cannot seem to feel God's presence, I will hold on to this revelation. When I am so deep in the valley that I cannot see the top of the mountain, during those times when I feel completely alone, I will realize that they are just life's clouds that are passing between me and my God.

The presence of the darkness does not indicate the absence of God, it is during these dark and lonely times that He is working hardest for us. Even Job, the man the Bible calls "most faithful," questioned God's presence during his trials and tests. (Job Chapter 30) We must remember that during these times we must walk by faith and not by sight.

We must get to the point in life where we relinquish negative thoughts and persons who are holding us captive to negative thinking. We must realize that everything is temporary and therefore we should not treat temporary challenges or conditions, or even friends, as if they will last forever.

Everything passes. Whether we receive healing or we pass into eternity, nothing remains the same. So do not give a temporary situation more power than it deserves. We must exact everything out of today rather than missing today's blessings by focusing on tomorrow's potential worries, or worse, yesterday's issues.

There will be persons who, each time they see you, they present pitiful countenances, even tilting their heads to the side when they ask, "how are you doing today?" If you say, "I am doing well," their retort is "are you sure?" They are convinced that once you are down, you will stay down. They seem to prefer a negative response rather than a positive one.

You must let go of these negative persons. They will always "bring you down." More often than not, you will be depressed and discouraged after speaking with them. They will leave you empty of everything good. Rather than encouraging and uplifting you, they will constantly remind you that you are battling some type of difficult challenge. They will try to get you involved in a pity party. Remove them from your life. Your survival depends on your attitude. Be hopeful. Be cheerful. Hold on to God's promises.

This morning I telephoned my friend who has the bone cancer. His wife answered the phone. That was unusual because he always answers the house phone. After some pleasantries I asked to speak to him. "He is very weak and in extreme pain," she explained. "He can only chat for a minute." When he said "Hello" I knew that he was very ill. After a couple minutes, she took the phone from him and said, "although he would love to chat more, he is too ill and needs to save whatever energy he has to get through the day." She and I chatted for a bit and she said, finally, "He is on his last lap"

That was the last time he and I spoke. Overnight he died quietly, in his sleep, at home. He always wanted to die in his sleep, at home. He had multiple carcinomas and far outlived the doctors' expectations. To the end, he fought a good fight and never, ever lost faith in God. He had said, some weeks earlier, that as long as he lived, he would continue to praise God, no matter what, and when he died he looked forward to living with Him in heaven. He felt, either way, it was a win/win situation.

He told me the week prior that he had lived a good life. He admitted that he was stubborn but that was all in the past. He bragged that he had the prettiest wife in town and two awesome, and now quite successful, children. He was a proud grandfather of a precious baby girl. He felt that he had "done it all" and was very grateful to God for all His blessings. My only response was, "Amen!"

LOOKING QUITE GOOD ON PAPER

Following the recommendation of the medical oncologist, I went to see my surgeon to check out the possible reason for the intermittent pain in the lower left side of my abdomen. The surgeon ordered an upper GI CT/Pelvis with contrast scan.

I am in the radiology room of the Hospital and the Technician says, "We will give you four containers of solution to drink. Wait ten minutes between each drink. We will return in forty minutes."

Forty-five minutes later, the scan began. Thirty-five minutes later I was on my way home.

A week later I returned to the surgeon's office. Once again, he is pulling on his beard while reading the report. He then circles a paragraph and says, "You are looking quite good on paper." "What does that mean, Doc?" He said, "Everything is looking great, there is only one small area along the colon wall, that is showing some possible sign of inflammation but, overall, there is nothing to worry about. Your appendix has already been removed. It is not a hernia or anything like that, so it must be a slightly torn ligament, as we originally discussed." He gave me a copy of the results, a prescription for a round of antibiotics and suggested I take some pain killers if it persists, "but there is nothing to worry about"

Everything sounds great, I think. At least I am "doing quite well on paper."

Remember the expression "bedside manners?" When we were children, each time we visited a doctor, we mentally graded them as having, either good or bad bedside manners. Of course, it had nothing to do with actually being by one's bedside, but rather the manner in which the care professional treated you.

This was determined by the way they listened (or not) until you finished your complaint, the way they explained (or not) in layman's terms, what exactly was the matter and how the treatment was going to be handled. A smile, some eye contact, some empathy, anything and everything that related to how respectful and caring (or not) your visit was handled, was referred to as a doctor's "bedside manner."

I cannot explain what I expected today. Although I really like my surgeon, I would have preferred him saying, "The tests came out quite well, I think everything is going to be just fine" instead of "You are looking quite good on paper." That expression seems quite open ended. It was as if, although the results indicated that everything was fine, maybe something was not outlined on the paper. I decided to let it go.

Many health care professionals appear to be so involved in research, financial gain, their own life goals and other personal interests, the personal touch and bedside manner have all become dinosaurs of the past.

When I was much younger, small town doctors knew your name when they walked into the office, even before they opened your file. They recognized and acknowledged you in social settings, outside the office environment. Granted, my surgeon is one of the nicest persons I know, but he can surely benefit from a few classes in how to translate what is on the paper into "patient's language."

The next day, I took the Report from my handbag and read it. I read the circled paragraph. What was really strange to me was that it noted "The uterus is not enlarged." "Really, I asked myself?" My uterus was removed almost twenty (20) years ago, so how could it show up on the scan? As well, the area of mention (on the lower right-hand side) related to the appendix. My appendix was removed the same time my uterus was removed. So how is it that they are showing up on the scan? Very strange, very confusing and a bit troubling. I sent an e-mail to my surgeon before I went to bed asking the above questions and I anxiously await his response. This will be quite interesting.

He is so wonderfully efficient. He responded early the next morning stating that the electronic reports are produced from a report template which, although convenient for details, gives the radiologist 'adjustment options' in interpreting the report to be able to specify in each case what the particular findings are and adjust the language of the findings. So "the uterus is not enlarged" translates, in this instance, to "no uterus was seen." He also explained that the report did not say "appendix." It said "appendices" which referred to representations of fatty tissue which normally extend from parts of the colon. Apparently, there can be any number of these structures along the colon wall and they may become affected by disease processes.

"Not to mention those findings on the report, would have been misconduct and malpractice on my behalf" he said. The whole response sounded complicated, but I understand what it means and I am satisfied with his response.

At times, our mind can be a weird mechanism, if I can call it that. I know the Bible says the death and life are in the power of the tongue, but the quotation from the Bible which I think all cancer patients and survivors should put up in front of them daily is: "As a man thinketh, so is he!" "Guard your heart and guard your mind," we are told in the Good Book.

Isn't it amazing that although, thanks be to God, everything is on the mend and all of my tests have come back negative, still the slightest new pain breeds fear in me? This phenomenon is common in the lives of cancer survivors, who, after having gone through so many challenges and in some cases, having been misdiagnosed at the outset, are always overly conscious that another serious problem may present itself at any time.

Although, since I last visited my surgeon, the pain on my left side has been negligible, I have now been experiencing some pains in my head. I would not refer to it as a headache, as there are about three different types of pain periodically. Normally, I do not worry about head pains because I was a sinus sufferer for most of my adult life. But these pains seem to come from the center of my head as well as the base of my skull, and sometimes, at the same time.

Once again, off to the doctor I ran. Thoughts of brain cancer tried to fill my psyche, but I kept reminding myself that all the recent tumor markers were well within range. Once again, I turned to my God. I fully believe that God has healed me from all my diseases and forgiven all my sins. One comes with the other, Jesus died for both, so if I believe for one, I must believe for the other.

Now that the surgery and radiation are behind me and being satisfied with the lower abdomen diagnosis, I realize that my faith is now my biggest battle. I know that with God on my side, Jesus in my camp, and the Holy Spirit interceding to the Father on my behalf, I will win this faith battle as well. As you can imagine, however, having been misdiagnosed twice, my human self is constantly bombarded with the "what ifs," so I have to constantly grasp tightly on to my life giving and lifesaving faith in God.

The ENT doctor, who knows my cancer history, examined me. He was quite aware of my fears, although unspoken. After a thorough examination of my ears, eyes, nostrils and throat, he quietly and gently stated "Everything is O.K. there is nothing *sinister* going on in there, just some sinus buildup and a bit of infection in the cavities." He explained that the pain in the center of my head is related to the sinus buildup and the pain at the base of my skull could be related to the osteopenia. Isn't it amazing how our minds play crazy tricks on us? Shortly after the doctor told me that "nothing sinister" was happening in my head, the pain virtually disappeared. He prescribed medicine for a period of ten days and said to take all of it in order to completely clear up the infection and any residual discomfort.

Mind over matter, big time! I think it boils down to the fact that cancer is a very scary and potentially life-threatening disease. Because in many cases, it either just creeps up on you or is misdiagnosed for a time before it is discovered, every pain or ache puts us on edge.

About six months ago, I was really encouraged by a commercial put on by a local breast cancer group. It was encouraging women, in general (and men who are breast cancer sufferers/survivors) to join a support group to benefit from the support and knowledge that is available from other longer-term survivors. The lady in the commercial said, "Once you hear the stories of other survivors, you feel much more confident in the knowledge that not every pain indicates another cancer battle."

She explained that cancer and the related treatments hurt for a long time post-surgery and usually there is no reason to be unduly concerned every time you get a pain or an ache, once you are submitting to your regularly scheduled follow up visits with your doctor and carefully following their advice.

I have attended three meetings so far and the information is really reassuring and informative, but human nature prevails at times. I strongly suggest that every cancer patient/survivor join a support group.

It is very important to get regular checkups and to "know your body" as well as having an in-depth knowledge of your family's medical history, so that each pain and ache does not constantly throw the fear of cancer or some other possibly fatal disease into your face. Many times, over the years, I have attended doctors for problems that seemed to stop on the way out of the office. Mind over matter. Once you get that official assurance that everything is O.K., suddenly the pain is no longer "life threatening." Isn't it amazing?

LIFE HAPPENS . . .

October has dawned and I have very much to be grateful for. I am happily celebrating one year being in remission. To God be all the glory! I am pleased to report that it has been eight months since my daughter, who was with me during the surgery, secured another job, which she loves. I am extremely happy for her and her family.

It is almost ten months since my son has been "seeking his passion" which translated, means unemployed. We no longer discuss it when we speak, but I continue to pray for him daily and I truly believe that God will deliver him from this enormous mistake he has made. He moves from friend to friend's apartment. At this rate, he will soon run out of friends. It is very disconcerting and embarrassing to me and our family. His sisters, who have him and his son over each Sunday for dinner, are very upset with him (although they contain it for my sake). They are angry with him because in these financially tough times, he made a conscious decision to leave his job. What was he thinking?

We are each afraid to "take him in" as he has nothing to bring to the table and only heaven knows how long it will take for him to find employment. Besides, everyone is in their own struggle right now and cannot afford the extra expense of an obviously selfish and unthinking young man with a big appetite who loves to watch sports on TV. Dollar signs ring out in our heads when we think of him living with us, although I think my younger daughter gives him handouts sometimes. They were always extremely close.

I redirect my thoughts to prayer whenever he pops into my mind, which is more and more, recently. It is very worrisome, especially not knowing how diligently, if at all, he is trying to find employment. I pray incessantly and will continue to talk with God until He sees fit to bring this whole fiasco to a finish. I need God's peace in this matter so I will continue meditating and singing myself into the light. I am confident something good will happen soon.

I just received an e-mail from a friend with this quote:

I believe in the sun, even when it is not shining, I believe in love, even when I do not feel it. I believe in God, even when He is silent.

I have no idea where the quote originated, but it is what I needed this morning. I fully believe in God and know that this too, shall soon pass. I will do my part and hold on to His promise of that peace "that passes all understanding" and His promises for my children.

November rains have begun to cool us down a bit. I go for walks to the beach and not have to worry about getting all sweaty by the time I return home. I love the fall evenings here along the Florida coast.

My son called today, asking to "borrow" some money for a bus ticket to New York City where he says he has a job interview. According to him, "It's a sure thing." What do I do? If I do not give him the money, I will always wonder if he would have landed the job, had I provided the opportunity. I cannot live with that weight on my shoulders.

I decided to take the chance and send the funds to him. I told him that my cash flow was very low at this time and that the money I give him would be his birthday and Christmas present all in one. I included an extra $250 for incidentals. One week later and no word from him. I wondered if I should call him or wait. I waited.

He called the following day. "I got the job, I start on Monday." He was ecstatic. "I'm very, very busy getting set up. A friend of a friend is allowing me to live with him until I am able to find an affordable place." He thanked me again for the ticket money and the additional funds. "I would not have survived without it, Mum," he continued. "I am using the last of it to have my clothes dry cleaned and purchase a new pair of shoes for the first week of my 'new life'. I want to make a good impression."

He went on to say that he was very ashamed of his impulsive decision to leave his secure job to try to go into business for himself, without giving it enough thought or having enough funds to get any viable venture off the ground. He was embarrassed that he had to bunk around with his friends and set a bad example for his son. He especially regrets that now he will be so far away from his son, but promised to visit as often as possible and hopefully relocate back home after establishing himself in New York. He vowed to do everything possible, to "catch up" with his responsibilities and pledged never to put me through such worry again. He actually cried. Of course, I cried, too.

I told him that this "drought" period in his life could have been God's way of fully convincing him that before he makes any other irrational decisions, he should ask His guidance first. If he leans on God to guide him, he will never repeat this unfortunate situation which has not only impacted his life, but the lives of his friends, who helped him over the past months, as well as his family.

He said he was sorry he would not be able to come down for Thanksgiving. He has to begin saving towards getting a small apartment for himself, while assisting his friend with utility expenses. I understood. I did not criticize him or remind him of how much money he owes me for his son's support. I will write that off. I did, however, remind him of God's forgiveness and blessings and encouraged him to become closer to God through His word and fellowship with other Christians. He promised to find and attend a church.

To God be the glory! He hears and answers the prayers of the faithful. Prayer, sincere heartfelt, faith filled prayer is the answer to everything. We must give all our concerns to God, and even though we will continue to be plagued by the doubts that come to trap us into disbelief, we must immediately return to His word and His promises to us and respect His decisions and His timing.

Note to Journal: No matter the outcome, we must believe that God is always with us and has the master plan for our life.

I immediately called my daughters and gave them the good news; they were both very happy and relieved. My youngest daughter said, "I will send him a house-warming gift for his new place." I knew exactly what she meant. They both promised to spend time with his son, as often as possible.

I received a telephone call early this morning from my radiation oncologist's office saying that I had missed my last appointment. Since the surgery I still have three doctors following my progress so I guess it's not difficult to forget an appointment. But I think the receptionist forgot to schedule a follow up appointment the last time I visited the office. Since she had a vacancy today, that is where I spent my lunch hour.

As I usually do, whenever I go from one doctor to the next, I always photocopy any medical testing results that I received since the last visit. I carried her the Onco test results, the results from the Upper GI testing and the results received from my new primary care doctor for my annual physical. She read them and asked the usual "How have you been since you were last here?" I told her about what precipitated the tests results that I just handed her. I mentioned that although I underwent a mammogram and an ultrasound in July just past and it showed everything was great, I wanted her to check my right breast as it occasionally hurts, similar to how the situation with left breast began.

She gently rubbed her hand back and forth over the area, and after a while assured me that she, too, could not find any lump or any reason to be concerned. She examined the lymph nodes under my armpits and was pleased to find nothing to be concerned about there either. She agreed with me that it may be "referral" pains but she suggested that I continue to monitor it, just in case.

During the examination, when she moved her fingers under the left breast, I felt a sharp pain. She too, was taken aback. She then re-checked the area and suggested that maybe as a result of the fusion of the skin due to radiation treatments, a nerve ending might have been caught up with the flesh. She reminded me to be careful when dealing with the area. Scar tissue should eventually provide some relief. If her suspicions are accurate, I may have the discomfort for some time to come, whenever pressure is applied to the area. She apologized but noted that there are other alternatives that could have been much worse, which I totally agree with.

She concluded the visit by strongly suggesting that I begin a more defined, regular exercise regimen to improve my circulation, strengthen my upper body and ensure my blood pressure remains acceptable. She advised that endorphins released during exercise are invaluable to my overall well-being. To achieve this, in addition to my daily walking, I will join a gym to build up my muscles and further strengthen my bones. I keep being reminded that I am not yet out of the woods.

Well, another year of life has come and gone. Praise the Lord I am alive and healthy and able to celebrate another birthday. I feel great and I'm very happy and satisfied with my life. I usually take my birthday off from work, but because it falls on a Saturday this year, I took the Friday off and planned a long weekend of celebrations. I have so much to celebrate!

I began by celebrating with my (deceased) husband's sisters, who are still near and dear to me, even after all these many years. We "girls" went to a really nice, well known restaurant. We ate, drank and were very merry. We laughed and celebrated for almost three hours, making sure to compensate our waitress accordingly. It was an awesome evening.

My daughters are organizing the usual birthday luncheon for our family on Sunday after church and I am eagerly looking forward to it. We always have an absolutely fun-filled time together, especially with the grandchildren in tow.

This evening, which is my birthday, two of my childhood friends and I, with whom I go back almost forty years, but have not seen each other since before my surgery, are meeting at a popular steak house near me. I can eat steaks almost every night, but of course, now I save them for special occasions, like tonight! We had a wonderful evening. As usual, our first order of business was to "solve all of the world's problems." We then shared stories about our children and grandchildren, our aches, pains, our hopes, dreams and plans for the upcoming Thanksgiving and Christmas holidays. We had a lot of catching up to do.

I have not yet mentioned my "situation" to them, but this evening, inasmuch as it has been almost fifteen months since the surgery, I am now comfortable sharing with these "drama queens" and being strong enough to withstand and respond to the barrage of questions and comments that will follow.

Please understand that I have not yet shared with them because I could not handle any worry-warts disturbing my peace. I needed to be totally focused on my healing. Everyone is different and I cope better with the least distractions possible. In addition, we live in different cities, and we have different lives so I was able to avoid seeing them although we often chat on social media.

I waited until the end of the meal when we were all very relaxed to announce that I had something I wished to share with them. Of course, they did not know what to expect. I imagine they thought I found a new beau.

I told them how it (the cancer diagnosis) all started and what has transpired over the past two years. As expected, they were quite shocked at the news and it took a couple of minutes for them to digest everything. Then the questions began. "When did the surgery take place," "how come we did not know when you were so sick," "how come you did not tell us before," "how has it affected your finances, your life," etc.

I slowly recounted everything to them and then quietly explained that I was not emotionally able to speak comfortably about it until now. I described to them, my challenges, feelings and faith. I told them I needed to protect myself from "sympathy" and other similar emotions of those around me. I needed to go inwards and seek God's strength and lean on Him versus leaning on human strength and clichés. I told how, firstly, I had to wrap my own head around what was happening before I was ever in a position to verbalize to anyone else what was going on. They both teared up, as did I.

Just as I expected, the more vulnerable of the two jumped up from the booth and came around to me and gave me a big hug (for which I braced myself) and said "I am so, so sorry." "Sorry for what?" I asked. "I feel very badly for what has happened and that you went through so much of it alone," she said. I assured her that at no time was I ever alone. I explained, "That is the reason I did not share before, because it is vital to my emotional health that everyone treats me normally, not as if I am sick or sorrowful. I prefer you both to be happy that I have survived so well, rather than being sorry for me."

I told them that I truly believe I was chosen by God to experience this challenge and that I believe God has intentions for me to be a testimony to His healing, forgiveness and His promises for my life.

I pointed out that my chance for survival is no better or worse than anyone else's. None of us know what tomorrow will bring, so my goal is to enjoy my life, family and friends as if there is no tomorrow. I am determined to get 100 percent out of each day.

That helped them both to get back on track and we continued to discuss my journey to this moment. They congratulated me for being so strong and we thanked God for His answered prayers. I, however, could see their minds racing and realized that tomorrow I could expect telephone calls from them with more questions.

One of the girls, her husband is also a great friend of mine and he is famous for not keeping secrets. I begged her not to say anything to him . . . yet. I wanted her to wait until she calmed down. In the end, it was a fun, but draining, evening. It was not until almost 1:00am that I fell asleep.

My family and I enjoyed the church service and the potluck luncheon afterwards was fun. The grandkids played games and watched TV. The girls and I shared our hopes for my son's future and I brought everyone up to date on my latest doctors' visits and the state of my health. We had a light but delicious meal. It was the best birthday ever! I am so grateful for another year of life. They left around 4:00 p.m. so that they would arrive home in time to get ready for the next day of work and school.

Within an hour after my family left to go back home, my friend called. She begged me to allow her to share the news with her husband. She said that he would be very "hurt" if he found out that I shared with her and did not include him. This is exactly why I am so careful with whom I share this information, and while I realize it is difficult for a wife to withhold such information, I only wanted her to calm down for a day or two before letting him know. Now I can expect a call of reprimand from him.

You tire of people who sorrowfully and continually ask, "So, how are you doing today?" as if they expect something to have gone wrong since you last saw each other. This is completely counter-productive to our desire to remain positive. I hope that will not be the case with her and her husband.

Thanksgiving is now just three days away and most of the U.S. East coast is experiencing large thunderstorms with lightening and flooding. The media is forecasting one of the biggest cancellations of airline seats for Thanksgiving in a few years. Atlanta, Raleigh, N.C. and both New York Airports are virtually closed down.

Today is November 26, the day before Thanksgiving. I understand it is madness at the airports and on the streets due to the "winter storms." My children and I are wondering if it is safe for them, this afternoon, to drive almost three hours in the rain, especially because some roads along their route experienced high wind conditions overnight.

I have not seen so much rain since Sandy wreaked havoc along the East Coast last year. It is quite dark outside and it is only 11:00 in the middle of the day. Very unseasonable. As I continued to look outside the office window at the ominous clouds, the sky seemed to be closing in on me. I smiled to myself as I compared the sight to one of my colleague's mood swings; at times dismal and ominous and then the clouds blow away, and she is again on top of the world. It is remarkable how each day brings a new and different challenge.

I am disappointed that the weather has cancelled my plans to go for a quick walk this evening after work. I really want to be consistent because my radiation oncologist told me to increase my exercise regimen and while I have gradually begun to do so, the pain in my lower left abdomen still "bugs" me, occasionally, when I exercise. "Should I worry about it," I asked myself, after all my surgeon did assure me that the upper G.I. MRI, which were done early last month, showed that everything was fine.

I will continue with my regular exercise and weight training and pray about it. I will leave it with God and if I feel led to, then I will re-visit my surgeon and request a colonoscopy, just in case. My feelings of doubt, are being compounded,

I think, by the dark clouds and the non-stop, torrential rain outside the office window, which now seems to be blowing sideways. I am quickly coming to the conclusion that I will be spending Thanksgiving by myself this year, and most of all, will not be able to see my grandchildren. No one should travel in this weather.

An hour later my older daughter called me with the latest weather forecast: The rain is now moving quickly away from her city and eastwards from our coast, out to sea. It appears they will be able to make the trip, even if they have to delay the drive a couple of hours.

I am reminded that, like the weather, everything passes, just hang in here for a while. Thankfully, we were let off from work an hour early. I rushed to the Supermarket and began my last-minute Thanksgiving shopping.

We had the most perfect Thanksgiving, except for my son's absence. But his son came along with my older daughter's family, which was totally awesome. We skyped with him and took lots of pictures and shared them with him, that made him happy. The heavy rains were replaced by a noticeable dip in temperature, which was very welcomed. We were pleased, especially because this Christmas promises to be as warm as last year, so we fully enjoyed the nice, cool weekend.

> **Life Lesson:** When in doubt, reflect on the past and remember
> that nothing lasts forever, everything passes. Patience and hope
> are the keys. Just wait . . . things always have a way of working
> themselves out.

YET ANOTHER CHRISTMAS

Three Christmases ago, I was very apprehensive; in fact, I was downright scared. I was worried about what was happening under my breast. It now seems like many, many years later. So much has happened in the meantime, so many lessons learned, so many experiences lived through but most of all, my faith in the Almighty God is constantly renewed and strengthened. I tell daily of His mercies, His grace and His hand of healing on my life. He is real and His promises are real and relevant to me.

I am now entering into another phase of my life of giving back to humanity through words and deeds. My biggest lesson learned along this journey is that of humility. I can do nothing on my own. I have to seek God's guidance and His wisdom in everything I do. He alone has the master plan for my life. Nowadays, I only make tentative plans. Between where I am now and where I hope to go, I will enjoy every minute of the "ride." I have learned to appreciate everything around me so much more than before.

When I awake in the mornings, I inhale the clean, sweet air that fills my home. I revel in the fact that I can open my eyes and see everything around me. I listen to the birds chirping outside my bedroom window and my favorite blessing is that I can get up and walk to my window, open the blinds and see God's glory once more manifested in each beautiful sunrise.

I do not "suck my teeth" and complain that I have to go to another day of work; rather I thank God that I still have a wonderful job to go to and I am committed to doing my absolute best each day for my employers.

I am grateful that I have a closet full of beautiful clothes and I can choose whatever outfit I feel like wearing for the day. I always look forward to enjoying long relaxing showers and revel in the luxury of the warm, soft, caressing feel of my fluffy towel afterwards.

I am very thankful that I can go to my refrigerator and choose whatever I wish for breakfast and that I can sit down and enjoy it while relaxing and watching whatever program I wish on TV or, sometimes listen to an inspirational CD.

I am thankful mostly for God's hand of mercy and grace on my life and that I have the daily opportunity to freely and boldly call on His name and declare His goodness to everyone I come in contact with; that I can brag of my blessings and encourage others in their walk, wherever it may be taking them.

My priorities have changed a great deal over the past four years. I now laugh more, worry less, sleep better, and do not scold myself for being human, at times. Most importantly I take absolutely nothing for granted. I love my God and I love my family. I love every minute I spend with them.

Love is the foundation of my life—it is all about love for family, friends and humanity, in general but most of all, love for my awesome God and His faithful love for me.

Love. There is no better subject on earth. There is no more meaningful message. No song can truly express it, all the dictionaries together cannot properly define it and no truth can outweigh it.

Life Lesson: I am nothing, without God . . .
but with Him, I am and I have everything.

My Christmas celebrations were wonderful. I drove up and spent the entire week with my family. I always enjoy the long drive, although my kids do not like the idea of me being on the road alone. The grandchildren were overjoyed to show me their rooms, projects and games. We had a great time and the best part was that my son was able to spend two days with us.

We ate, we laughed. We shared our New Year's resolutions and even made diary notes to encourage each other to stick to them, which most likely we will not, but it was fun anyway. Our New Year's celebrations were also very enjoyable. We went to church around 11:00 p.m. on New Year's Eve and then we went out for a light meal afterwards. The evening was wonderful. All around us, we heard fireworks and, in some instances, saw them as they lit up the sky.

I am so happy and grateful that God has spared my life to see another year.

Earlier this week, two distant friends of mine, died very suddenly. What a shock. The younger one was only thirty-four and died in her sleep. Until the autopsy is released, everyone believes it was weight and grief related. She was obese and was still mourning the loss of her baby just a few months earlier. She never seemed to have gotten past her grief.

The other friend, forty-three years old, went in to have her appendix removed and within a week of being discharged, she died. Why? I doubt if we'll ever know the real reason.

Each day above ground is truly a blessing. Death is no respecter of persons. Any sex, any age, any health condition, rich or poor, it does not matter.

I am ready for all the blessings, knowledge, wisdom and courage God will bestow on me in this new season of my life. Isn't it amazing how after being diagnosed (with anything life threatening) each holiday, birthday, anniversary, in fact, each day is so much more of a blessing and a gift to be treasured, than pre-diagnosis?

The weather up along the east coast is rainy and very cold, but here in Central Florida we are still relatively warm for this time of year. I do, however, look forward to a "touch of cold weather" later this month so I can wear my fluffy sweaters and light jackets. They always make me feel like I am engulfed in a warm hug. I hope that some of the cold comes our way, albeit not all of what is happening up north.

Back to reality now that the holidays are behind us. I am working long hours because our company's year-end is December 31 annually, so the first few weeks in January are always very hectic with deadlines to complete various Reports to allow the external auditors to "take over the books" before the official year end results can be released. It is an incredibly stressful time but once it passes, things settle back into some form of normalcy.

The pain in the lower left side of my abdomen never quite disappeared and my tummy has been a bit upset these past weeks, although I chalked it up to the holiday festivities, but today I decided that this must end. I have made an appointment with my surgeon to get to the bottom of this. It has been going on for far too long now.

Both my surgeon and my medical oncologist assured me that "everything is fine" when I visited them with this same pain in August of last year when I had the upper GI and all the tumor marker tests done, so why am I still having the pain and why are my bowels now misbehaving, to boot? My tumor markers last month were all within range and I am still celebrating that victory.

I remind myself that we, all, must take some personal responsibility for our health and our life. Only God is God, not the doctors. I thought about dismissing the pain, but when my forty-three-year-old friend died after being rushed back to the hospital post-surgery, I rethought it. Her family and the doctor are still in shock because nothing was seen to be potentially fatal during or after the surgery. No one is able to understand what went so wrong, so fast.

Too many times and often too late, it takes autopsies to reveal the real problem (that the doctors were unable to diagnose). Let the doctors regard you as a hypochondriac, do not concern yourself, that is a small price for your good health and peace of mind. Besides, you are paying for the service and health insurance is not free, so I decided to return to the doctor to get a satisfactory answer to what is happening in my lower abdomen.

Remember, too, it took eleven months of my insisting to the doctors that something was wrong, and two mis-diagnoses before I was correctly diagnosed with breast cancer. In the meantime, it had progressed to Stage 2 (into the lymph nodes) despite there being an actual, obvious, sizeable indentation on my breast.

If I have to visit five doctors this time, I will not stop until I have a satisfactory solution to the problem. While I accept that the deaths of my two young friends may have something to do with the urgency of my decision, I will not overthink it or let it overwhelm my thoughts. I realize that there are always two voices in my head—one positive and one negative, it is like the commercial with an angel on one shoulder and a devil on the other.

Although the voices of fear and negative thinking seem to be trying to take over right now, I will continue to talk myself into a positive attitude. I remind myself that death and life are in the power of the tongue and all thoughts begin in my head, so I constantly repeat God's promises to me and the one that I repeat most often is "I can do all things through Christ, who strengthens me." My colleagues here at work often laugh at me because they hear me mumbling, but hey, let them laugh, at least they are laughing at one of their existing colleagues—not a former colleague. I will, however, stop the audible mumbling as I know it is distracting.

> **Note to Journal:** I remind myself that "this battle is not mine, but the Lord's" and I will sit back and observe His victory.

I will not verbalize any negative thoughts, no matter how strong the urge is, no matter how obvious the condition is, I will continue to glorify God and His perfect will for my life.

I am now in the doctor's examination room, being handed the, now all too familiar, paper gown with the split at the back. Have you ever wondered why the split is in the back, especially when you are visiting the doctor regarding an issue that is in the front, in which case you have to take off the gown and expose everything anyway? I can never understand it. I decided to go against the status quo and I put the split in the front, so when he examined my breast and abdomen area, all I would have to do was open the gown.

Oh well, the nurse asked me to remove it, anyway, and covered me with a sheet. So here I am again, being probed and pressed and listened to . . . and more probing and pressing and then, of course, the puzzled look that my doctors always seem to have on their faces when examining me. After the examination, I put my clothes on and return to his office.

Once again, he pulls on his beard while writing notes in the file. He then looks at me with a bit of a wrinkled brow and says, "I do not see anything that can be a cause for worry. I am forced to conclude it must be scar tissue from a previous surgery. I suggest, if you wish, you go and see a gynecologist just to be on the safe side and then return in five months for me to do your annual check-up."

He referred me to a gynecologist whom I had never heard of before, but who turned out to be one of the most efficient and caring medical professionals I have ever met. She was young and thin and very casually dressed. Although my initial encounter with her was not too much to my liking; she had to leave me there and go "just around the block" to pick up her kids from school, I was determined to keep my cool and I am happy that I did. She apologized profusely and explained that it was an emergency. The person assigned to do the school pickup, fell ill.

She appeared too young to be a specialist but once we got into conversation, I realized she was highly intelligent and apparently quite experienced as well. She began by asking me lots of questions, threw out some possibilities, and performed a thorough examination, including an ultrasound. She had her nurse set up an appointment, at a nearby laboratory, for me to have another scan done and a mid-way urine test. She prescribed three sets of medicine. She advised that it would take about one week for all the test results to come in and when they were ready, her office would give me a call, which they did.

A week later the results revealed a low grade, long term bladder infection, with a trace of blood in the urine and a tiny bit of fusion in the bladder and bowel area, possibly from a hysterectomy done many years ago. She said, "This can be corrected by a simple surgical procedure that should take less than an hour. I will prescribe some medication which should clear up the infection after about two weeks." She assured me that it was not at all life threatening, but something that should have been attended to some time ago. "Excluding the weekends, you should only require ten days recovery time."

I am more than ecstatic, even though I have to undergo the surgical procedure, more than a year of suffering will finally come to an end. I am also comforted by the fact that this whole thing was not just "in my head" and that I can now go on with my life without always wondering "what if." She arranged to have the procedure done the following Friday. Now I can begin planning the summer vacation I had promised my grandchildren.

Lesson learned: Never give up or accept advice about your health that you are not completely satisfied with, because only you know what you are experiencing inside. The extra time and dollars are all worth it . . .

A PERFECT LIFE?

Each one of us, whether cancer patients, cancer survivors, young women or old men, black, white or yellow, experience periods of drought, fear, disappointment, pain, loneliness and hurt in our lives.

We all, at some time were hoping for a positive result, a nod, some gratitude, a phone call from a loved one, a return on an investment. We have all sat by the phone waiting for a return call for a job interview, an acceptance from a college, something, anything, that did not happen. People have let us down, in fact, in many instances, we have let ourselves down, but just like any drought, it will not last forever. We must hold on to that thought when the pains come, when the doctor's report comes back a little scary. When friends disappoint us or we find ourselves unemployed, we must realize that nothing remains the same. While most times, life carries us in a positive direction, other times things may go south, but nothing ever stays the same, ever.

There is a saying that goes "Into every life some rain must fall" and while this usually refers to a problem or disappointment, this can also be the case when there is a drought of peace, happiness or health in our lives, we must remind ourselves that some "healing rain" will fall in time.

We must stand on God's promises to us and never waiver. It is not that God does not answer our prayers, it is us who do not patiently wait and believe and do our part in the meantime. We put a time frame on His response and when our self-imposed time frame expires, we then take matters into our own hands or worse, just give up entirely. This year, let us quiet our minds, be still and patiently wait for His response.

I believe that this year will be filled with happy rain, and although I am convinced of it, I am still aware that there will always be periods of drought in one area or the other of my life—nothing is ever perfect, nothing. When our health is good, we are always complaining about our finances or our relationships. Always some area of drought. We expect everything to be perfect at all times. Everything is relative and we, humans, complain entirely too much.

In order to move ahead we must accept reality. Accept that we will never have the total balance or control we have always hoped for and dreamed about. After all, many of our problems are from sources outside of ourselves and totally out of our control, i.e. mother nature, the global economy or relationships, whether personal or business.

We must never own the struggles, never personalize them, they are not ours to keep, nor are they here to stay. They are only here to grow us, once we learn the lessons therefrom. I have never said "my cancer" I have never owned any challenge. This battle is not mine; it belongs to God.

Be a faithful warrior, right until the end. The Bible says that with God, all things are possible (but it has to be according to His perfect will for our lives). My dear departed friend always said, "I will praise Him while I live and with my last breath." He was well aware that this earthly existence is only a chapter in our life, not the entire book. I have no idea how long I will reside here on this earth, but I do know that I have no intention of going out angry at God.

I know that no matter if my residency is only for a few more weeks, or for twenty more years, I will use every hour of every day to be the most joyful person I could be and I will sing God's praises from the center of my being until my last breath.

I will do my best to ensure that my children want to emulate my life and my tenacity and that my grandchildren speak of my wisdom, courage and faith in God until they themselves pass on.

Life Lesson: Know that God has already equipped us, through His word and His Holy Spirit, for every challenge or test He allows us to go through. Let us "gird up our loins" and go forth and watch God win this battle for us.

Almost five years later, I am again standing by the kitchen window sipping a cup of tea and looking out at the purple and orange sunset, enjoying the chill of the breeze blowing through, remembering that day, some years ago, when I first discovered the lumps in my left breast. The pane of glass is no longer missing, it was replaced just before Hurricane Sandy.

What a ride, what a journey through pain and fear, discouragement and uncertainty; hope, patience, courage and faith. The tears, disappointments, surgeries, the smiles, the laughs and the rewards, have all brought me to this day. I still have a way to go before I am declared out of the woods. I still have to check my tumor markers and other blood work every six months. I still have the occasional pain in my rib cage and my armpit. At times, I suffer side effects from the medicine. I still cannot wear my regular bras and I still have to take special care of my health, but I am now intentionally happy, realizing how much of a gift each day is.

I try to pass along my joy to everyone I meet. Instead of losing my temper or being impatient, I acknowledge that everything passes and it is not worth hurting my emotions and my body with foolish deeds or words of persons who are determined to be unhappy. I have come to realize that, in essence, we are all the same. We are all carrying some baggage.

Never, ever think you are alone. Everyone is fighting a personal battle of some sort. People are either going through, or will face, some disappointment, pain or suffering. We are all striving to be happy and accepted by those we love and admire. We are all seeking that illusive perfect life. Each of us, no matter our status, race, color or nationality, are all the same inside.

Each morning when I pray, I ask God to help me be a better person than I was the day before, filled with a strong determination to be at peace, grateful and empathetic of those with whom I come in contact.

I intentionally decide to make great memories as often as possible as these memories become the most sustaining gifts when we are "down and out," in pain, or need to put a smile back on our face. We can always encourage others with some uplifting anecdote. We can always go into our memory bank and pull out a few of the great memories we have enjoyed over the years. Immediately we are transported to another place in time that was filled with happiness and great memories.

So much has happened, so many changes have taken place in and around me. It seems more like a lifetime rather than five years. The old spiritual song says, "Through it all, I have learned to trust in Jesus, through it all I have learned to trust in God, through it all, I have learned to depend upon His word."

I have met and am now a part of so many other people's lives who have gone through this challenge with me, most of whom I have been able to encourage and uplift. I am grateful to my doctors, nurses and other medical team members who have provided such wonderful care over the years. I thank my faithful pastors on whom I have relied for prayers and intercession.

I thank God daily for my children, their spouses and my grandchildren. I am quite aware of the burden they quietly carried during my illness. I am grateful for the friends who stayed at arms' length, without constantly reminding me of my condition, but were right there in case of need. They, along with the many life experiences have caused a re-invention of the person I used to be. I am now a much humbler, forgiving, understanding, charitable, grateful and happy person, free from so many of the worries of the world that I now realize I cannot control. I now understand and accept that only God knows my tomorrow and He is already there preparing the way for me.

I am definitely not the person I used to be, nor am I yet the person I will eventually become, but I love my "now" and will revel in it. I do not know if the cancer will return, but neither do I know if a large meteor will strike and eliminate the earth next month, but today I am happy and healthy.

Today is the best day of my life. I have never been this blessed, I have never been this grateful, I have never been this age before. I have never been this smart, I have never been this happy with life and I have never experienced today before now.

Join me, let us both enjoy the marvelous gift of today.

MY GO TO SCRIPTURE VERSES

Psalms 23

Philippians 4: 4-7

Psalms 103: 1-12

Psalms 91

John 3: 16

Romans 8: 11

1 Corinthians 10: 13-16, 18

About the Author

Caroline Isador is a Christian who loves God more than anyone or anything in her life. She leans on Him for everything and gives Him all the praise and honor that is due Him. He is the reason she lives, and words cannot express her gratitude.

Caroline is a cancer survivor undergoing treatment and doing bloodwork, including tumor markers, regularly to ensure the medicine does not have adverse side effects or cancer has not spread to any other organ.

She is a mother and grandmother and spends as much time as possible with her family, who she loves dearly. Caroline realizes what a gift they all are and enjoys being with them and sharing her life and faith.

She wrote ***Living with Cancer: My Healing Journal*** to share her journey with anyone going through any life-threatening health challenge and attest that you are never alone. There are millions of others also facing similar battles in their life. Be assured that God is with you and willing to help you if you call on His help.

She is an executive assistant to the senior VP of a marketing firm, and grateful for her job and looks forward to going to work each day. Her favorite hobby has always been reading and researching various subjects to enlighten her knowledge of the world and the people who inhabit it. Caroline resides in Central Florida.

www.ingramcontent.com/pod-product-compliance
Lightning Source LLC
Chambersburg PA
CBHW070118030426
42335CB00016B/2196